# MASSAGE

## for Healing and Relaxation

### Carola Beresford-Cooke

*Photographs by Nick Adler*

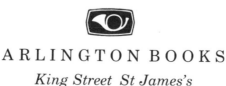

ARLINGTON BOOKS

*King Street  St James's*

*London*

*To*
*Clare Maxwell-Hudson*
*with love and thanks*

**MASSAGE**
*for Healing and Relaxation*

First published 1986 by
Arlington Books (Publishers) Ltd
15–17 King Street, St James's,
London SW1 by arrangement with
Thames TV.

Second impression July 1986

Third impression September 1986

Fourth impression September 1986

Fifth impression November 1986

© Text Carola Beresford-Cooke 1986
© Photographs Arlington Books 1986

Typeset by Inforum Ltd, Portsmouth

Printed and bound in England by
RJ Acford Ltd, Chichester, Sussex

British Library Cataloguing in Publication Data
Beresford-Cooke, Carola
Massage.
1. Massage
I. Title
613.7′9      RA780.5

ISBN 0–85140–690–4

**For Thames TV:**
Researcher: Lesley Hilton
Director: Christopher Bould
Producer: Valerie Brayden
Series Producer: Nina Burr

# CONTENTS

# INTRODUCTION

Massage, the oldest of the healing arts, is enjoying a new revival, moving from its traditional domain in the beauty salon or sports centre to take its place alongside the newer healing therapies. Professional massage treatment now comes under a variety of labels – reflexology, Shiatsu, Rolfing, bio-dynamic massage, pulsing, Touch for Health and many more. Its unique value in soothing the mind as well as healing the body is now widely recognized. But the practical uses of massage in treating common complaints encountered in everyday life are not yet widely known.

I feel that massage need no longer be the prerogative of the professional, but that it should take its place in the home as an aid to family health and as a means of relieving the increasing stresses of daily life, with all its attendant illnesses. It is a skill, certainly, but one which is very easy to learn and to apply, particularly where there is already a bond of affection between the person giving and the person receiving.

The aim of the Thames TV series *Massage* and this book is to make massage more accessible, with application to everyday family situations. Tense shoulders, arthritic hands, the aches of pregnancy, a child's cough, a torn muscle: all can respond to this easy and pleasurable home treatment. Indeed babies are happier when they are massaged, and couples can literally smooth out their conflicts, while old people feel comforted and cared for. All the family can benefit from massage, and you may only wonder how you will find the energy to do it all!

In fact, massage need not be tiring. I have stressed in the explanations of the basic strokes that massage is done not with the hands alone but with the whole body. Try to think of your hands as flexible, feeling extensions of your body, and keep them utterly relaxed, so that they mould themselves naturally to the shape of the area you are working on, while the power of the movement comes from your back, hips and legs. Massage given in this way becomes a swaying dance which invigorates instead of tiring you. Your hands, instead of straining stiffly and conscientiously to 'work at' the massage, become two magic antennae which pick up signals from your partner's body. Always trust your intuition, do not follow the book blindly (although there are a couple of warnings you should not ignore) and do not be afraid to invent your own strokes and variations. There is no such thing as 'correct' massage – everybody's style is unique, which is the beauty of it. Your massage is an extension of *you*, as lovely to give as to receive; so try it, and enjoy it!

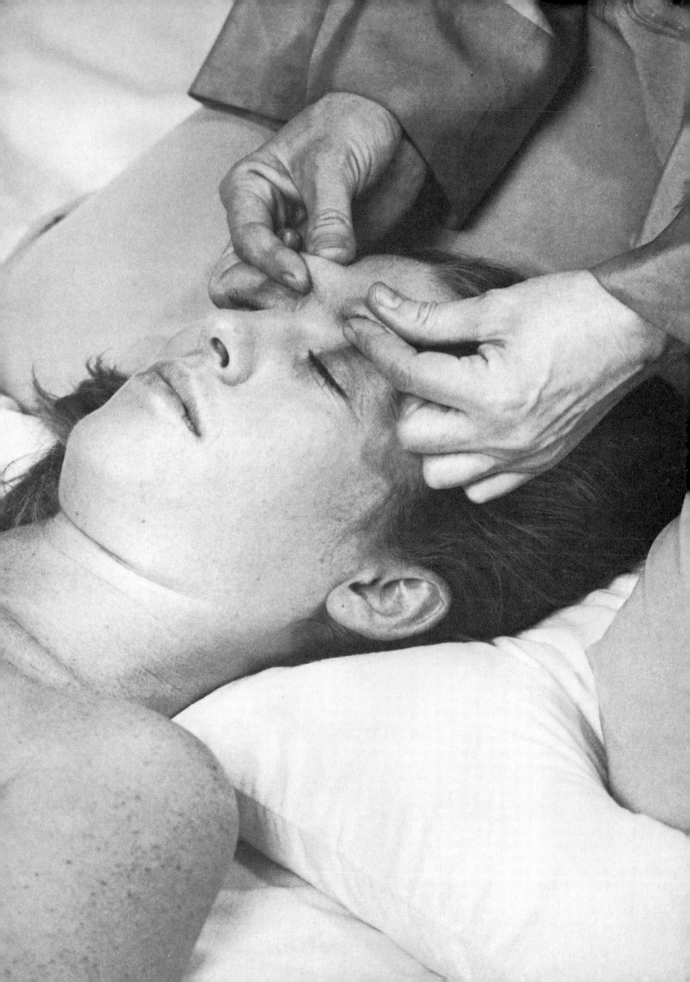

## The shoulder rub

The shoulder rub is the most welcome form of massage you will ever give. Most people carry tension in their necks and shoulders, often because of bad posture or occupational hazards such as sitting for hours at a typewriter. Tense muscles cause pain and stiffness, deprive the brain of circulation and may result in fatigue, grogginess and headaches. A good shoulder rub will relieve these symptoms and leave the person massaged feeling brighter, perkier and more relaxed. You do not need oil, and your partner does not have to remove any clothes. It is also an excellent way to start learning massage. Make sure your partner is sitting comfortably and upright, remove any jewellery and undo tight collars. Now you are ready to start.

1. First, place your hands gently on your partner's shoulders. Remain completely still for a moment as you channel your thoughts towards your partner and take a deep, quiet breath. Be very aware of the touch of your hands on her shoulders. This gentle contact sets the tone of your shoulder rub and begins your partner's relaxation process.

2. Squeeze the shoulder muscles gently but firmly, moving from the neck outwards, several times. This takes the contact further, and allows you to feel the areas of tension in the muscles.

3. Holding your partner's forearm with one hand and holding the shoulder on the same side with the other, take her arm slowly in a circle, forward, up, back and down. Do this two or three times. This is 'passive exercise', loosening the joint, gently stretching the ligaments and tendons and increasing the circulation. Take the arm in as wide a circle as is comfortable, but do be careful not to force it or over-extend, especially if at the beginning there was any pain in the shoulder. Changing hands, repeat this movement on the other side. *(Below)* Repeat it as many times as you like in

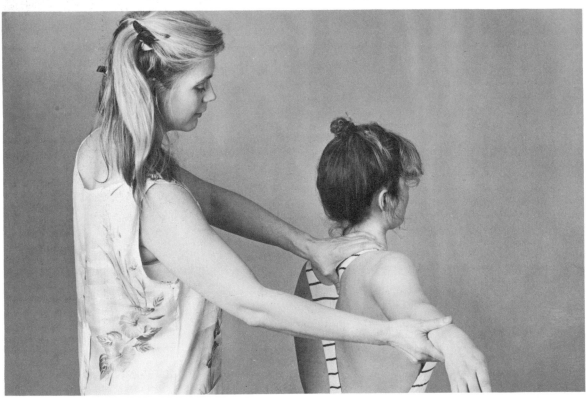

between the other movements in the sequence. You will find that the arm moves more freely as you progress.

**4.** Placing both hands on your partner's shoulders again, move your thumbs in tiny circles up the edge of the shoulder-blades. Do this quite deeply but without causing pain to your partner. This movement is called 'circular frictions'. It is very useful for detailed work on areas of muscular tension – tiny circles for specifically knotted areas, larger circles for more general stiffness. Continue up the muscles at the back of the neck, down again and across the top of the shoulders, and anywhere else your partner complains of tension.

**5.** If your partner's arm is held horizontal and slightly back, you will see a hollow at the back of the shoulder joint. This is a trigger point to release the muscles of the shoulder. Locate this point on both sides with your thumbs, and press gently but deeply for a few seconds, or until there is a release of tension. (*Right*)

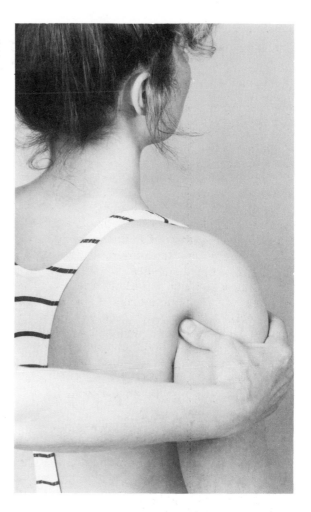

**6.** With your elbows loosely bent (that is, not in a sharp point) lean gently on the top of your partner's shoulders, on a spot about halfway along the muscular ridge. Increase the pressure gradually as if you were leaning on the back of a chair. This spot is sometimes painful, but your partner should feel a release of tension. Lean for a few seconds. (*Below left*)

**7.** Support your partner's forehead with one hand, so that her neck is relaxed. With your other hand, work up the neck muscles with a circular squeezing movement, your thumb on one side of the neck and your fingers on the other. Try to make the movement deep but without being painful. It helps to imagine that you are reaching *inside* your partner's neck to soothe away stiffness and tension. (*Below right*)

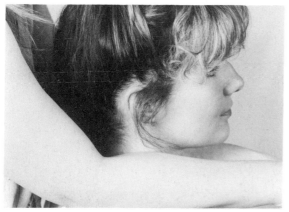

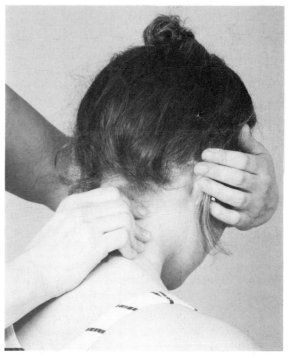

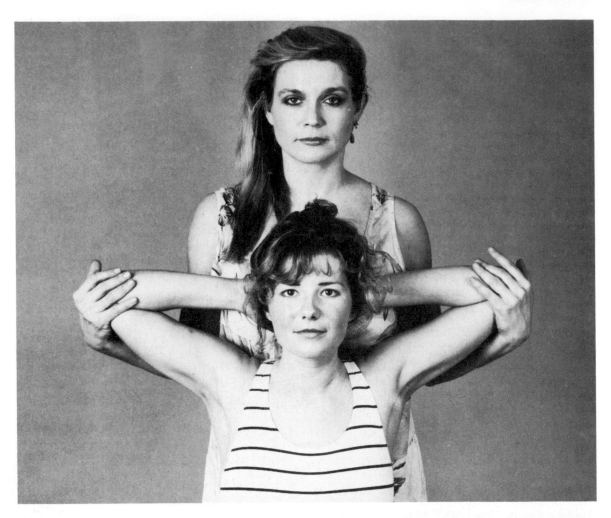

**8.** Just under the base of the skull at the back of the neck, in a hollow halfway between the centre and the ears on both sides, is another pressure point. Pressure here is good for relieving headaches and colds, as well as stiff necks. Place your thumbs in these hollows, and with your fingers on your partner's temples, tilt the head back and press gently upwards with your thumbs, so that you stretch the neck and stimulate the pressure point at the same time. *(Right)*

**9.** The Stretch is a final relaxing touch. Ask your partner to clasp her hands lightly behind her neck, and gently take her elbows backwards till she says 'stop'. Hold this stretch for a few seconds, then replace her arms gently in her lap and squeeze the shoulder muscles again with the lightest of touches. *(Above)*

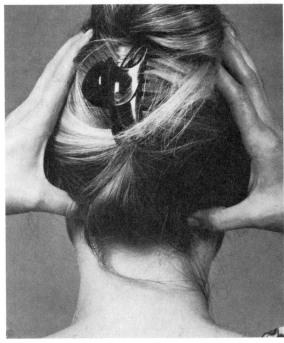

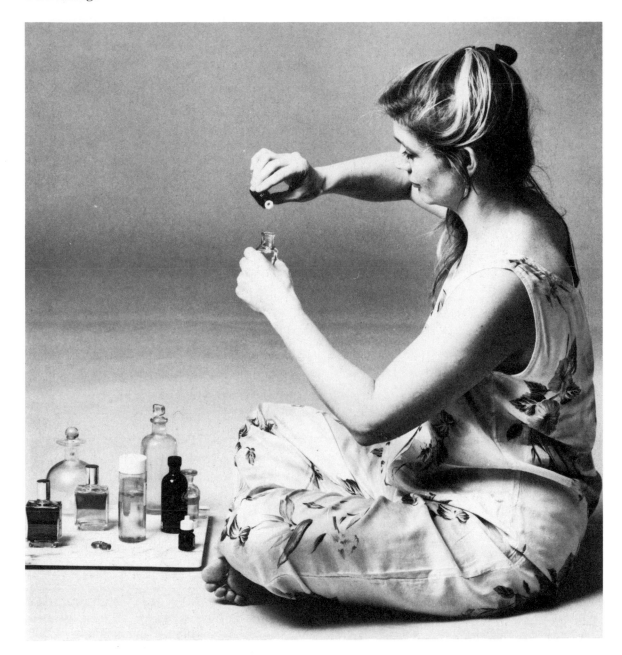

# Oil massage

To begin to appreciate massage as an art, you will probably want to begin working on the body as a whole, and for this we usually use oil. Massaging with oil allows your hands to flow smoothly over the skin and develops *rhythm*, which is one of the best natural tranquillizers for the body, mind and spirit.

When preparing for an oil massage you will need a comfortable surface for your partner to lie on. I use a towel over a quilt on the floor, but a table is fine if it is the right height and padded with blankets and towels. I do not advise a bed; for one thing, it is too low, and gives you backache, and for another it is not firm enough to provide adequate support.

Have the room very warm, and keep extra towels and blankets handy to cover your partner. When you lie relaxing without much clothing on for any length of time you can get extremely cold, so make sure all the parts of your friend's body which you are not actually massaging are covered.

Any emollient oil or cream is suitable,

## ESSENTIAL OILS

| | |
|---|---|
| *Camomile | – inflammation, stomach irritation, tension, insomnia, aching muscles. |
| *Lavender | – pain of any kind, tension, insomnia. |
| Rosemary | – poor circulation, fatigue, chilliness. |
| Geranium | – swellings, up and down moods, diarrhoea, water retention. |
| Sandalwood | – dry skin, urinary infections, tension. |
| Ylang-ylang | – insomnia, tension, fast heart-rate. |
| *Clary Sage | – lower backache, problems of the female reproductive system, childbirth. |
| Juniper | – toxic conditions, painful joints. |
| Lemongrass | – aching muscles. |
| *Melissa | – depression, insomnia. |
| Marjoram | – painful joints, cold feeling. |
| Peppermint | – painful joints, hot feeling, indigestion. |

*These essential oils are suitable, in dilution, for use by pregnant women.*

although obviously some are better than others. I prefer oils of plant origin, as they are better absorbed, and benefit the skin. Almond oil is odourless and fine-textured – Indian grocers often stock it fairly cheaply – but sunflower oil, with its slightly nutty smell, is a good second choice.

Scent adds a further dimension of pleasure to an oil massage, and natural herb and flower essences are in themselves therapeutic, as well as smelling delicious. They penetrate the skin very quickly to reach the bloodstream, and are thus a wonderful adjunct to massage therapy. Essences are very concentrated, however, and should never be used undiluted, or they may irritate the skin.

Aromatherapy, as the use of these essences is known, is becoming increasingly widely known and practised, and there are many good books on the subject, some of which are listed in the back of this book. Among the most useful and relaxing of the essences for the beginner are lavender and camomile; you might want to add some ylang-ylang or sandalwood for extra depth of scent. Add two or three drops of the essence of your choice to about half a teacupful of oil for a full body massage. Do not make up too much oil at a time unless you intend to do a great deal of massage, as it begins to smell 'off' after a while. If you do want it to keep, add some wheatgerm oil, to help prevent the oxidation process which causes the smell.

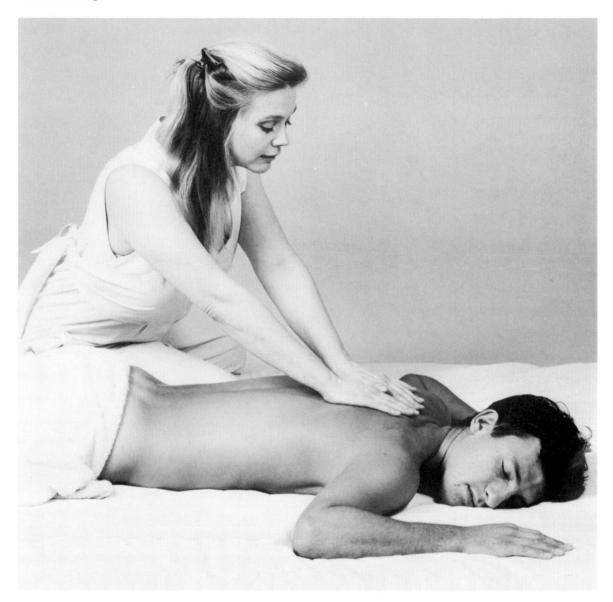

# Back massage

### The basic strokes

The back is a good place to begin learning massage techniques, for two reasons. Firstly, it is a large, flat surface on which to practise different strokes. Secondly, it is our central support and the core of our nervous system, and thus gets tired, tense and achey. Almost everyone suffers from some form of back pain or tension, and massage is an excellent way of relieving this discomfort.

*A word of warning, however. If your partner is experiencing acute back pain of recent onset,* *has suffered a serious injury or undergone back surgery, do not massage the back without first checking with a doctor.*

1. The first contact with your partner is the application of the oil. Pour about a teaspoon of oil into your palm, and spread it over the surface of your hands to warm it slightly. (If your hands are cold, do warm them over a heater or under the hot tap.) Never pour cold oil directly on to the skin – it feels horrible. Once warmed spread the oil gently over the surface of the back, from bottom to top, in long, smooth strokes. Do not dab the oil on the back.

2. *Effleurage. (Above)* The oiling movement can change imperceptibly into the first

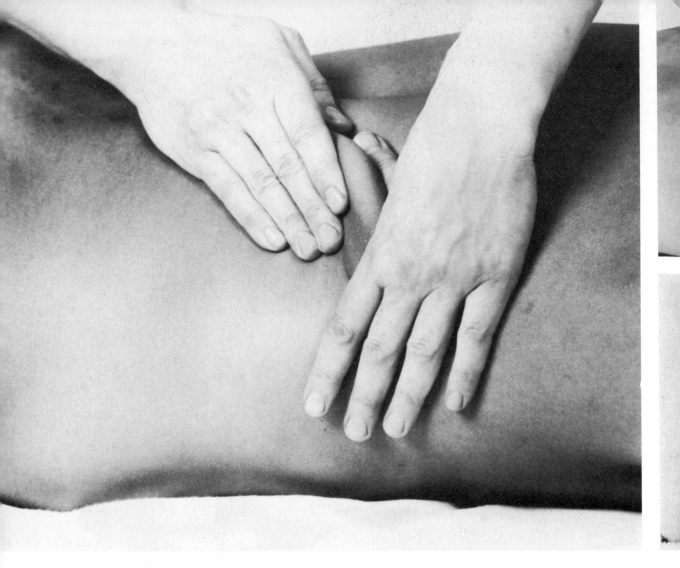

massage stroke which is called *effleurage*, a French word meaning 'skimming the surface'. Effleurage, in effect, works on the body surface, soothing the superficial nerve ends, toning the skin and above all making your partner aware of himself as a whole, rather than feeling like a head with some more or less useful – or uncomfortable – bits and pieces attached. Stroke, firmly but with relaxed hands, up both sides of the spine, and out across the shoulders to the top of the arms and gently down the sides of the back, then up again over the waist to the base of the spinal column to your original position. Repeat, so effleurage becomes a continuous movement, with the emphasis on the up-and-out rather than the back-and-down movement.

The massage will flow better and tire you less if you move from the hips, rather than the shoulders, so that you are using your whole body. It is essential to relax your hands so that they mould themselves to the body surface. Remember that rhythm in massage contributes to the relaxing effect; if you play some music during your massage, you will discover how it can help you find your own rhythm. Vary your effleurage occasionally with a stroke up the sides of the back, on to the tops of the arms again and gently down. Once you have established a rhythm with your effleurage, you can go on to the next movement.

**3.** *Petrissage*. This is the French word for 'kneading'. The movement does not much resemble kneading bread, though it feels like it from the receiving end! Face your partner's body and grasp a handful of flesh next to the spine in one hand. *(Above)* Squeeze it between your fingers and thumb allowing the oiled flesh to slide into your palm. As you let it go, pick up another handful very close to it with

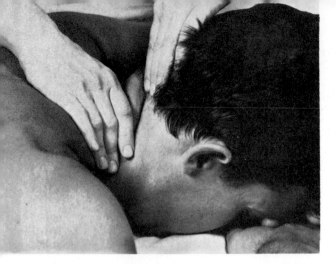

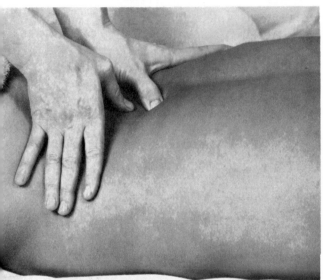

grain of the muscle and softens it, breaking up fat or lumpy tissue and improving circulation.

Follow your petrissage with effleurage to re-establish a rhythm.

**4.** *Circular Frictions.* As I explained in the shoulder rub (*page 6*), this movement is used for specific areas of tension, such as each side of the spine. It is done with small, penetrating circular movements of the thumbs, either separately or together, up the sides of the spine. You can use larger thumb circles over larger areas such as the small of the back or the shoulders as an alternative to petrissage – on thin people, for example, where there is not much flesh to 'knead'. This movement works on the nervous system, like effleurage, only deeper, to root out deep tensions – remember this when you do it, and make your movements 'seeking', penetrating ones; not hard or painful, but deep. (*Bottom left*)

Return to more effleurage, before moving on to try the most stimulating massage stroke.

**5.** *Tapotement.* In English this means 'percussion'. (*Below*) The best way to describe this stroke is to call it a drum roll up and down the back, made either with lightly clenched fists to

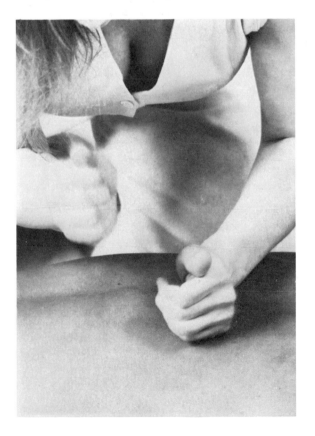

your other hand. Repeat, so that your hands are working in unison on the muscle, grasping and releasing alternately with a sliding movement. Now increase the rate, establishing a rhythm as you did with the effleurage. You should be using your whole body, rocking slightly from side to side. Now that your hands are working as a team, you can move them up the back, working across the grain of the long back muscles; turn your hands to knead across the top of the shoulders; then down the side of the back nearest you.

As you get more adept at petrissage, you can put a twist into it from the wrists, so that the movement is more versatile and effective. Petrissage can cover a large or a small area – try doing it using big movements and your whole hand on the small of the back, then with small movements of thumb and fingertips on the back of the neck (*Top*). It is done across the

13

relax the muscles or with the edge of the hands to tone them up. Just remember the drum roll, and it will give you an idea of the speed of the movement. It is important to remember that you must not do percussion directly on the spine. Practise on the edge of a table before you try it on a partner. This will show you how to work lightly as well as quickly. (You hurt your hands if you do not work lightly!) The most important thing is to keep your wrists relaxed. When tapotement is done well it feels wonderful, so if you find you have the knack (I don't!) do use it. *(Right)*

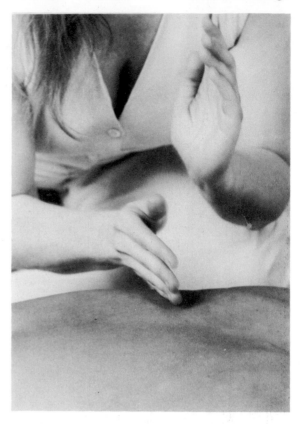

To finish your back massage more effleurage, the movement to which you frequently return like a familiar melody. Lastly, featherlight stroking with your fingertips and long strokes from top to bottom of the back, barely touching the skin, to soothe and hypnotize. *(Below)*

With this basic repertoire of strokes you can massage not only the back but also, with very slight adaptations, the whole body. Specific instructions for massaging the limbs, belly and face are found in the following chapters.

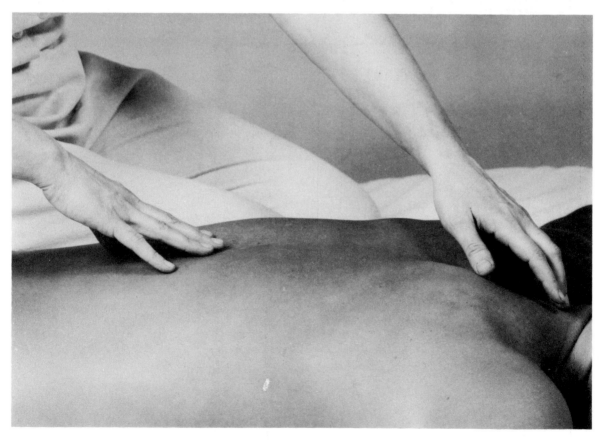

# SHIATSU

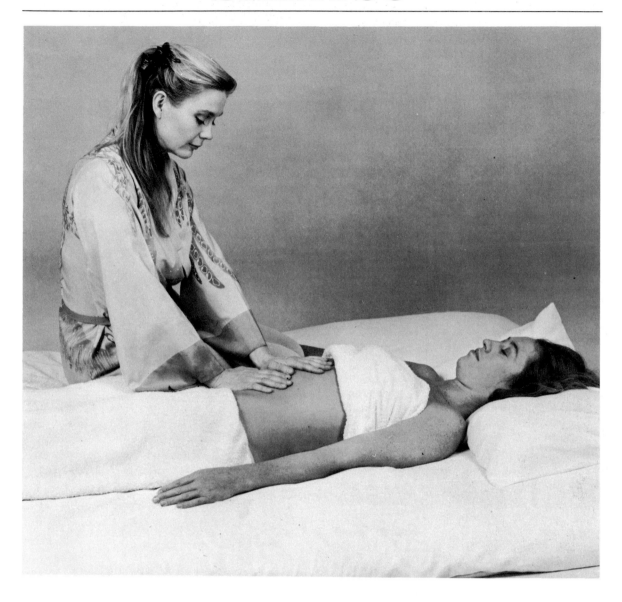

*Shiatsu* is a Japanese word meaning 'finger pressure'. It is the name of a style of Oriental massage therapy increasingly widely practised in the West, which is closely linked to acupuncture. According to acupuncture theory there are pathways of energy throughout the body, known as 'meridians', which influence the functions of the various organs. Along these meridians are specific points which can correct the balance of the energy flow, restoring health and well-being. Shiatsu is the art of applying pressure to the meridians and points.

No oil is used, and the massage is given through clothing, which has obvious advantages. No privacy is required, and you can give Shiatsu anywhere. Besides this advantage, Shiatsu is an extremely relaxing therapy, with a deep effect on all bodily systems. Given by a master, it is a powerful healing art, but even at beginner level it can help to prevent disease and relieve many minor ailments.

*But do use your common sense. If your partner has serious health problems, consult a doctor first; and if in doubt, do not give Shiatsu.*

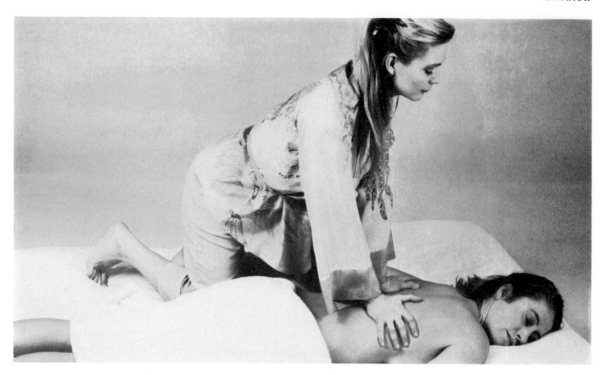

# Back Shiatsu

The first lesson in Shiatsu is the most important – 'do not press – be supported'. Good Shiatsu is not a proof of strength, but a very natural 'leaning' on your partner's body with your own body weight. It is essential that you be relaxed when giving Shiatsu, and this involves putting your concentration into your belly rather than your head or hands. Keep your knees apart so that your position is stable, move from the hips, keep your neck and shoulders relaxed, and your pressure will be deep but comforting. *(Above)*

When giving Shiatsu to the back, make sure that your partner is lying with her hands by her sides, so that her spine is supported. Begin on the horizontal part of the back, below the shoulders. Place the heels of your hands on either side of the spine, hands turned out and relaxed, moulded to the contours of the back. Ask your partner to breathe in and then out. As she breathes out, sway forward from the hips and allow your weight to come down through straight arms on to her back. Sway back on the in-breath, move your hands down an inch or so, and on the out-breath sway forward again, allowing your weight to rest once again on her back. Continue down the back in

this way, co-ordinating your pressure with her breathing. Control your pressure by swaying forward more for stronger pressure, less for gentler pressure, as for example over the lower back and kidneys. Keep going till you come to the buttocks. Return to the first position and repeat the process, keeping your neck and shoulders relaxed and moving from the hips.

This series of pressures, swaying from the hips, is the basic movement of Shiatsu.

# Back of legs Shiatsu

To work on the backs of the legs, keep one hand on the lower back and bring your body weight through the other hand on to the back of the thigh. Move down the thigh with repeated pressures, keeping both hands relaxed, and remembering to move from your hips. As you approach the knee, use less pressure, and virtually none over the back of the knee itself. Increase it again slightly as you move on to the calf, and wrap your hand loosely around the calf as you continue to move down towards the ankle. Cross over to the other side and repeat the process on the other leg, remembering to keep one hand stationary on the lower back – this hand should maintain a light but steady

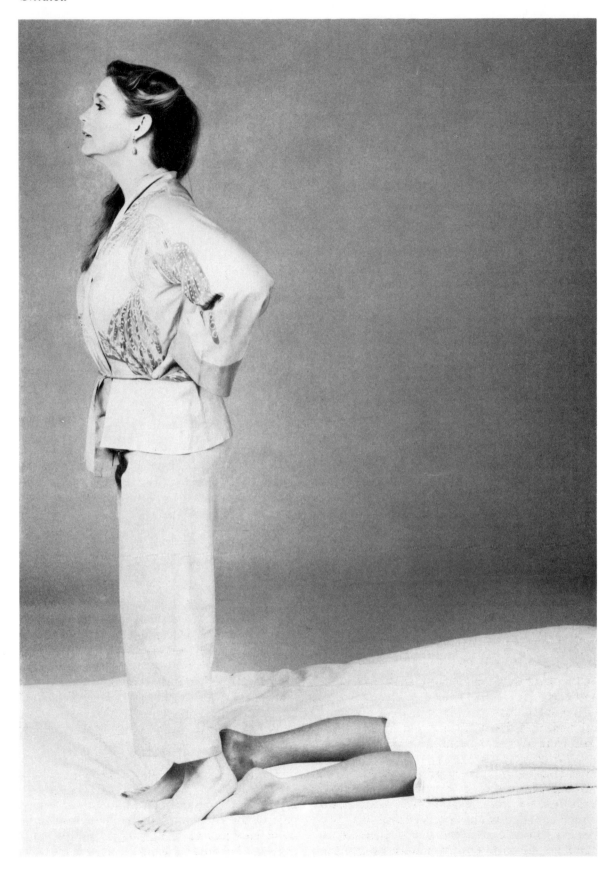

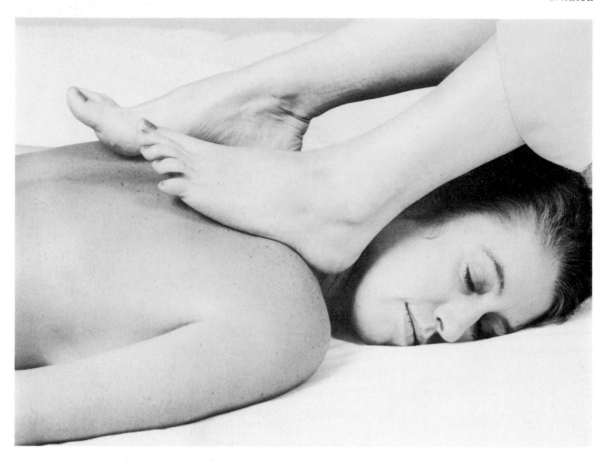

pressure as the other hand works gradually down the limb.

# Walking on the feet

When you have worked on both legs, make sure the feet are lying flat and, facing away from your partner, 'walk' on her soles. (Not everyone can do this – if your partner's feet will not lie flat, omit this movement.) Concentrate on the lower part of the foot – walking on the instep is painful. Do this for as long as it is comfortable to your partner. (*See previous page*)

# Shoulder Shiatsu

Move up behind your partner's head and sit, supporting yourself on your hands. Now place both feet on your partner's shoulders and 'tread' gently into the shoulder muscles. You can do this fast or slow, and as heavily or lightly as your partner wishes – experiment with different positions of your feet to gain maximum coverage of the shoulder area. It is extremely relaxing for your partner and very good for your legs! (*Above*)

# Face and head Shiatsu

Shiatsu to the face and head can be very useful in relieving the symptoms of sinus congestion and some kinds of headaches. It is also very relaxing, because we often carry a lot of tension in our faces. Your partner lies on her back, and you sit behind her head. Remember when working on the face that your pressure should be quite gentle.

1. Begin with the points at the inner corner of the eye-socket – not the eye – and press gently upwards with your index fingers for a second or two. (*Opposite top*)

2. With your thumbs, press on the thickest part of the eyebrow. This point is said to be good for relieving hay fever as well as sinus problems. (*Opposite bottom*)

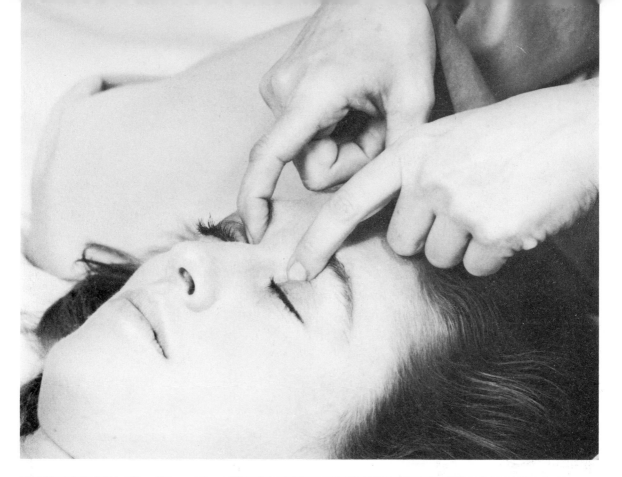

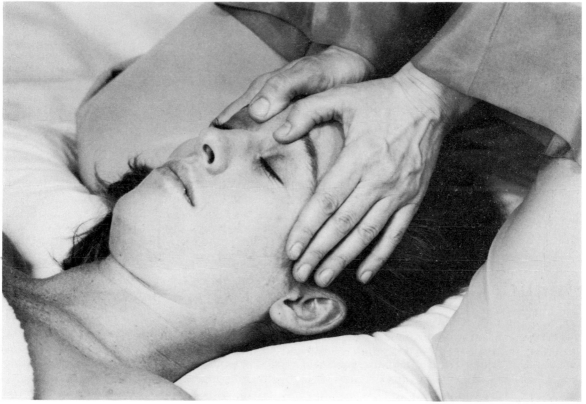

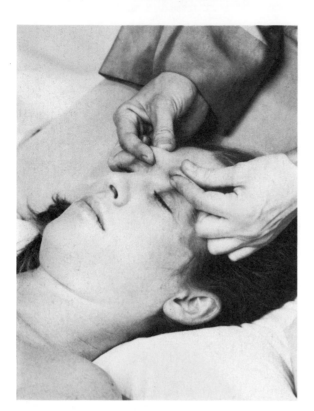

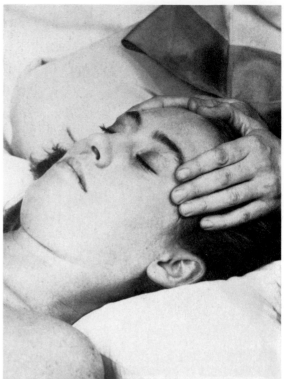

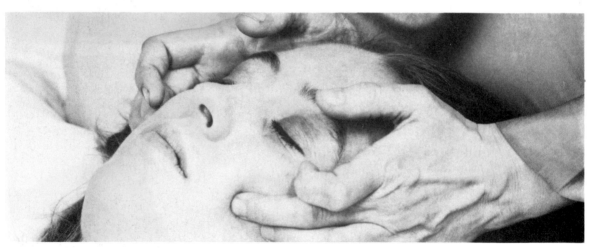

**3.** Pinch the eyebrows gently from the bridge of the nose outwards. *(Top left)*

**4.** Press gently with your fingertips on the temples and rotate slightly. *(Top right)*

**5.** Move your fingertips downwards to press into the hollow under the outer part of the cheekbone. *(Above)*

**6.** Press into the little knot of chewing muscles just within the angle of the jawbone. It should feel a bit like toothache to your partner. This relaxes tense jaw muscles. *(Opposite top left)*

**7.** With your thumbs at an upward angle, press upward and inward under the nostrils, to help clear a stuffy nose. *(Opposite top right)*

**8.** Press down the 'laughter lines', directing your pressure upward under the cheekbones. This helps blocked sinuses. *(Opposite bottom)*

**9.** Finally, overlap both your thumbs at the centre of the hairline, and press at small intervals back along the top of the head, checking with your partner that your pressure is still central. (It is easy to wander off the midline!)

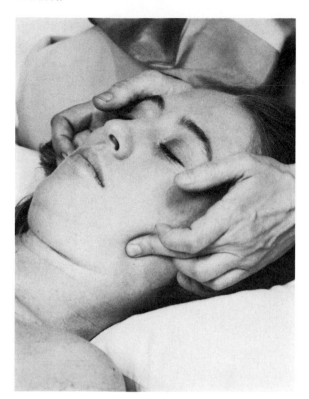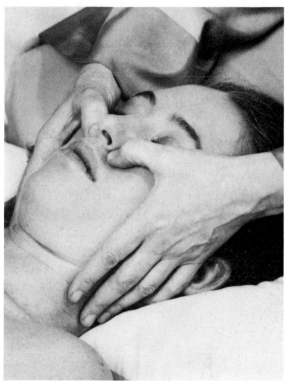

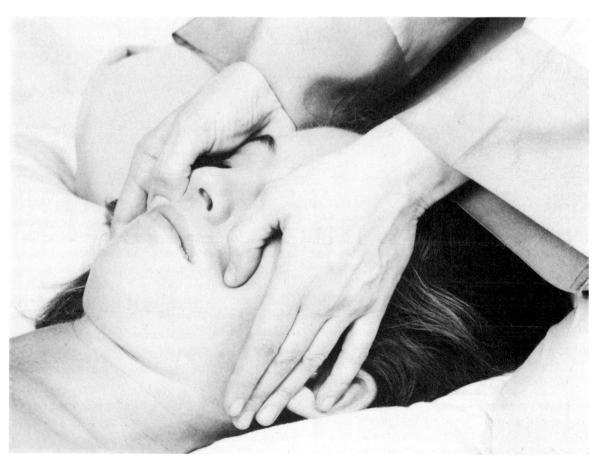

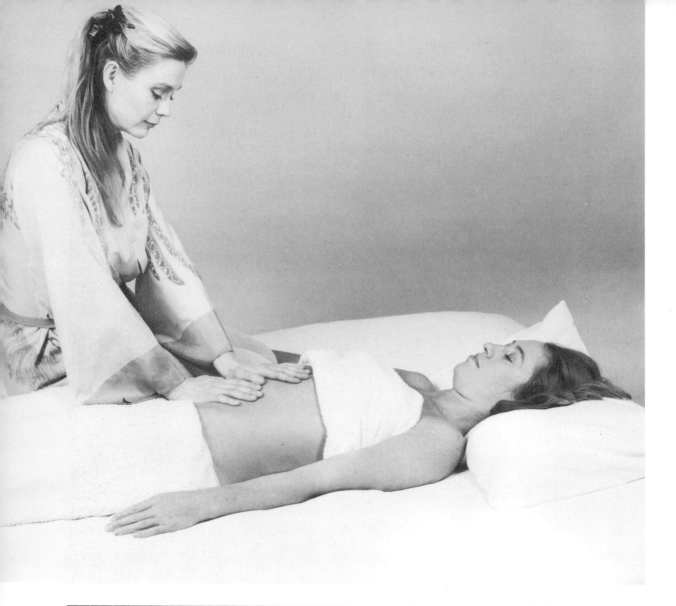

# Hara Shiatsu

Another area where the centuries-old tradition of Shiatsu can be very helpful is the abdomen, or *Hara*, as the Japanese call it. Shiatsu to the Hara is a very specialized art, and can be used to diagnose and treat all kinds of diseases, but even at beginner-level it can be useful for minor stomach problems, indigestion, constipation, menstrual problems and – surprisingly – backache. However, Shiatsu to the Hara should feel good. If the area is tender to the touch, do not work on it.

Begin by sitting comfortably, close to your partner, and rest both hands gently on the Hara for a moment. All touch here should be considerate and caring (although it can be quite deep) and you should always keep both hands on the Hara, one to work and one to comfort and 'listen'. For maximum benefit, you should work only lightly on areas that seem tight or tense, and concentrate upon parts which feel hollow, weak or soft. If your 'listening' hand picks up a pulse anywhere in the Hara, you should move to another area till the pulse disappears. Gurgles, on the other hand, are entirely a good sign!

**1.** Press the edge of your hand deeply into the area next to the hipbone. *(Opposite top left)*

**2.** With the upper part of your fingers, press clockwise around the soft part of the abdomen, once in a horseshoe shape around the outer edge, and again in a smaller horseshoe within that. *(Opposite middle)*

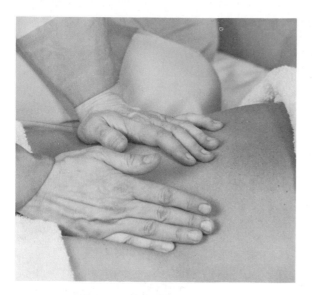

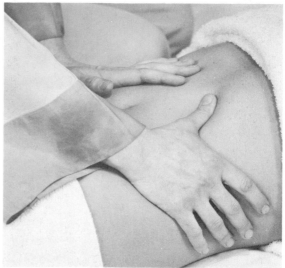

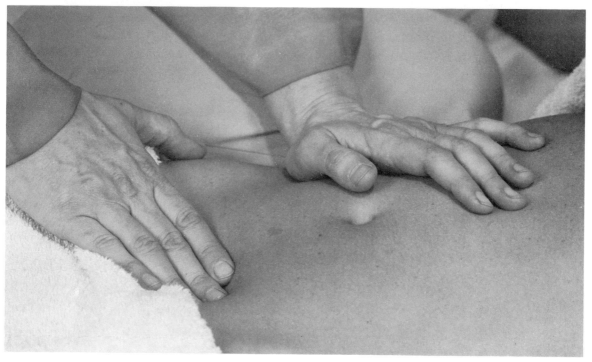

**3.** With the whole length of your thumb, press under the edge of the ribcage from top to bottom on both sides. The rest of your hand should be lying relaxed and moulded to the body while the thumb works. Let your partner tell you if the pressure is comfortable, and hold each pressure one or two seconds. (*Top right*)

**4.** Press gently with your fingertips in a line from the meeting of the ribs down to the navel. (It is quite normal to feel a pulse along this line, as the aorta runs under it.) (*Right*)

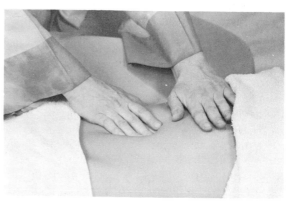

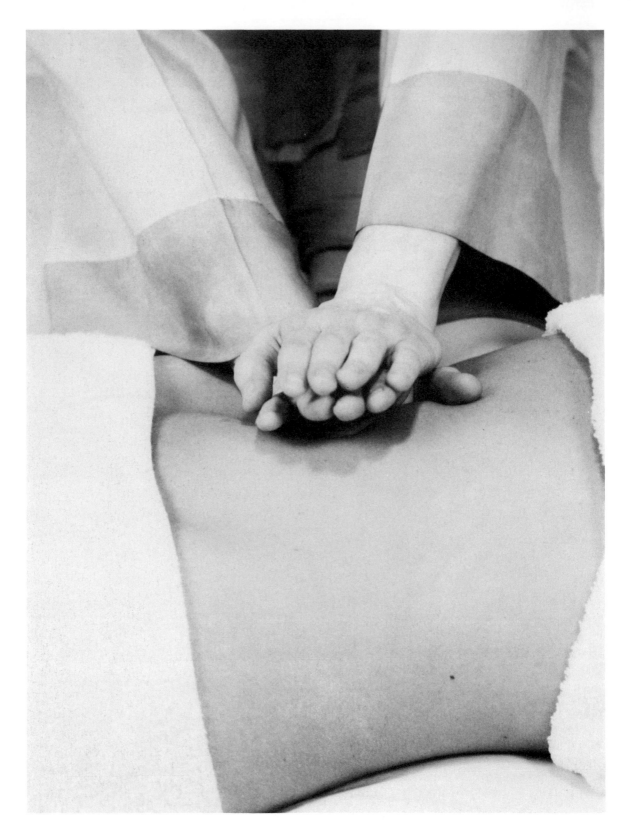

**5.** Finally, with one hand on top of the other across your partner's waist, rock the Hara by pushing with the heels of your hands and pulling with your fingertips. *(Above)*

# PREGNANCY AND BIRTH

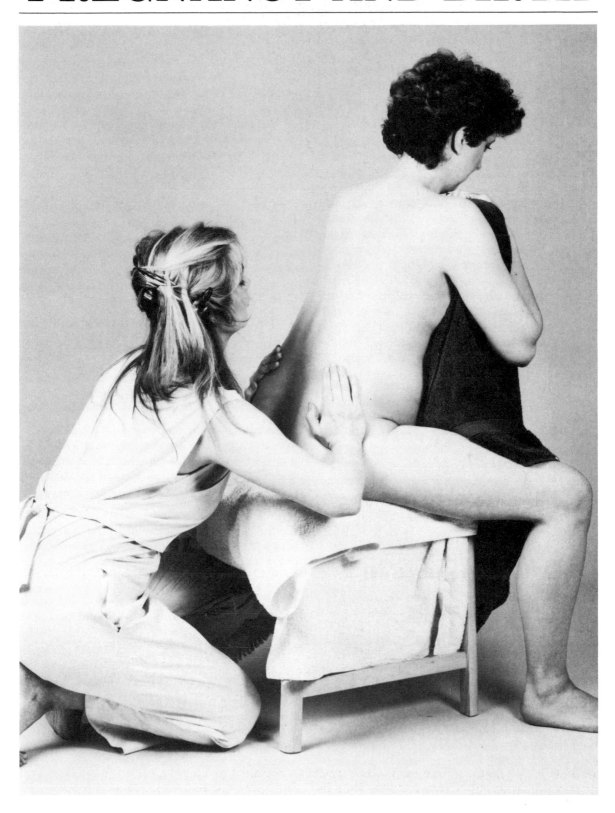

Massage is the most ancient form of folk medicine, and comes into its own during the months just before and after the birth of a new life, a time when other remedies, such as drugs, can easily upset the delicate balance of nature's processes. The aches and discomfort which sometimes accompany pregnancy, and the minor health problems of babies and young children, can often be avoided or safely treated by regular, gentle massage both of the mother and the baby.

# Pregnancy

Pregnancy involves an enormous adaptation of the woman's body, and this can sometimes cause discomfort. The main problem areas are the spine and its musculature, which must support an extra stone of weight at the front of the body; the legs, which must carry that extra weight around, and the abdomen itself, which must stretch to accommodate the growing baby. Massage can soothe and relieve aching muscles, improve sluggish circulation and, in combination with diet and exercise, maintain the body in good condition in preparation for childbirth.

However, there are certain precautions to be observed when massaging a pregnant woman. Be gentle at all times, do not dig deeply over the abdomen or lower back, and do not work on the legs if she has varicose veins. *If there is any problem with the pregnancy, or if the mother has high blood pressure or a history of miscarriage, do not massage without consulting a doctor.*

# Oils for massage in pregnancy

It is best not to experiment with essences during pregnancy. They are very strong, and may affect the baby. Stay with tried and tested essences which are beneficial to the womb: lavender, camomile, melissa, rose, jasmine – expensive but delicious, these last two! – are very beneficial during pregnancy, and may help to prevent stretch-marks. Lavender and clary sage are helpful during labour as a massage oil, as a compress, or even simply as a soothing scent to inhale. Always remember to dilute the essences in a carrier oil.

# Back massage in pregnancy

There are two positions in which to massage the back in advanced pregnancy, when the woman can no longer lie face downwards. The first is sitting astride a chair, leaning her arms on the back of a chair, which should be well-padded with towels and cushions. The second is the side-lying position.

### Astride a chair

**1.** After oiling the back with long, smooth strokes, give firm effleurage up the sides of the spine. *(Opposite top left)* Squeeze the shoulder muscles as you reach the top, and draw your hands gently down the sides before repeating the movement. Alternate with effleurage up the sides of the back.

**2.** Gently knead the shoulder muscles and the tops of the arms, as described in the petrissage section *(page 12)*. *(Opposite bottom)*

**3.** Relax tense back muscles with small circular frictions up the sides of the spine. Do not dig too deeply over the lower back.

**4.** Larger circular movements of your thumbs over the small of the back, around the buttocks and the bony triangle at the base of the spine will not only relax the back itself but also help to ease tension in the deeper pelvic muscles involved in labour.

**5.** Follow with gradual but deep palm pressure inwards on the sides of the buttocks to help relieve tension in the pelvic area. *(Opposite top right)*

**6.** After some more effleurage over the whole back, support the forehead with one hand and massage the neck with the other, as in the Shoulder Rub *(page 6)*.

### Side position

This position can be used not only in pregnancy, but also if there is any other reason – such as a stiff neck, or abdominal pain – why someone cannot lie on their front. It is a good position for deep work on the muscles of the shoulders and hips, and you can work on the legs in this position, too. If the woman crooks

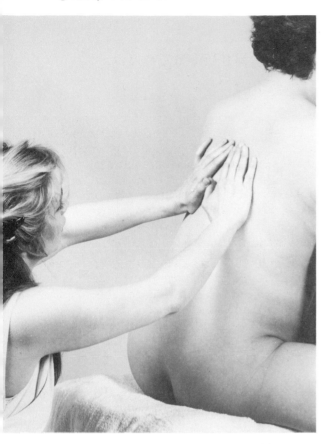

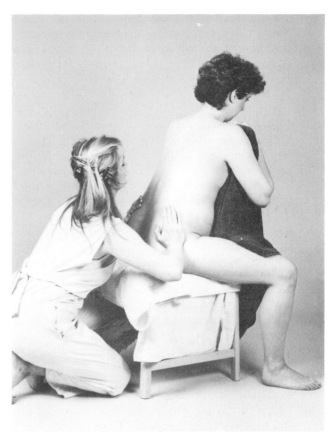

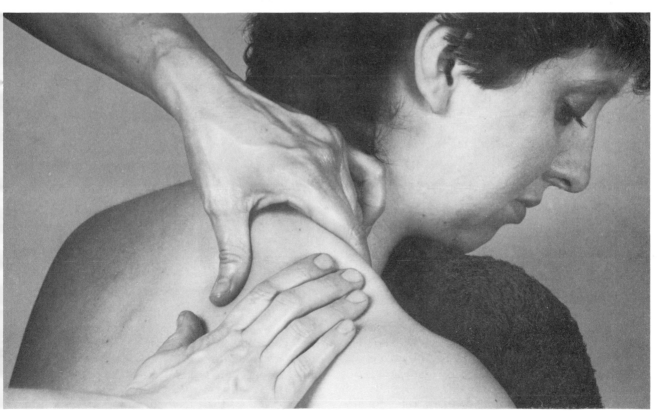

her top leg over, the position is quite stable and comfortable, and you can prop her up with cushions wherever necessary.

**1.** The strokes are much the same as in the previous position, except that you massage one side at a time. First, effleurage up the side, including the back, hips, ribs and shoulders. (*Top right*) Follow this with kneading on the shoulders and circular frictions up the spine, finishing with kneading on the neck.

**2.** A good movement in this position is deep circling, with one hand on top of the other, over the lower back, hips and buttocks. Keep your hands firm but relaxed, with most of your pressure on the heels of your hands. It is best if you can move the flesh slightly over the bone, rather than just making a slippery stroking movement, which does not do very much. Releasing the buttock muscles in this way also helps to relax the muscles of the pelvic floor, so it can be a good movement to do during labour, and especially in a 'back labour', when most of the pain is in the lower back. (*Bottom right*)

**3.** Effleurage on the legs encourages circulation and lymph drainage, often impaired by the extra weight-bearing of pregnancy. It is the same movement as effleurage on the back – firmly up, gently down – but remember to mould your hands to the smaller contours of the leg.

**4.** With wide open hands and relaxed wrists, make criss-cross movements across the thigh and the calf, to relax tight muscles. Effleurage over the whole leg again and then ask the woman to turn over. Repeat the whole process from start to finish on the other side.

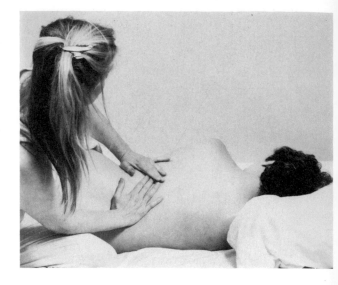

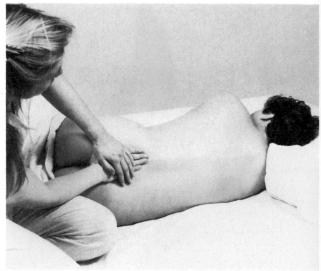

# Massage for abdomen and front of legs

Although many massage therapists will not touch the abdomen during pregnancy, a light massage here can be incredibly soothing to taut, overstretched skin and muscles. It can help prevent stretch marks, and, most importantly, communicates with the baby in the womb. So, when performing these strokes, try and imagine the baby lying under your hands, and that you are massaging not one person but two, as indeed you are.

**1.** After oiling the abdomen, do circular effleurage where one hand moves in a continuous circular motion and the other describes semi-circles around it. I was taught to do this in an anti-clockwise direction because this is the direction of the small intestine. Some massage therapists do it clockwise because that is the direction of the large intestine. I think we can conclude that the direction does not matter too much. What *is* important is to keep your hands relaxed and moulded to the contours of the abdomen. Do not press too hard! (*Opposite bottom*)

**2.** Without breaking contact with the abdomen, stroke up and out and around the ribcage, bring your hands down the sides of the back and round the hipbones towards the groin. Your pressure should remain firm but

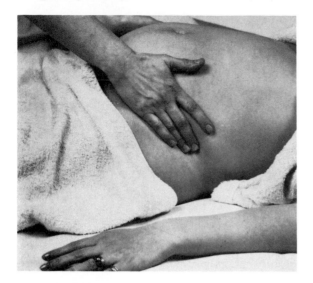

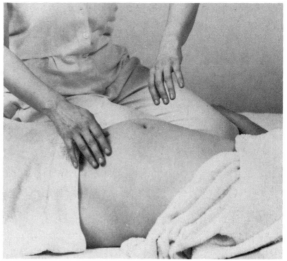

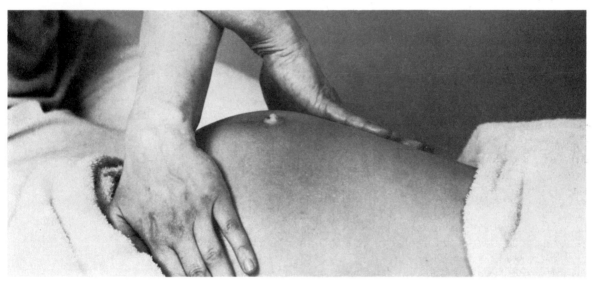

gentle until you reach the hipbones, when you use a lighter touch for the last part of the movement. Repeat and then return to circular effleurage. These strokes are the basic sequence for all abdominal massage. *(Top left)*

3. Another movement which some women have found helpful during contractions in labour is featherlight fingertip stroking downwards around the lower abdomen towards the pubic bone and a little way up on the other side. One hand follows the other in a continuous stroking movement, first on one side and then the other. The mother can do this herself during contractions, or her partner can do it for her. *(Top right)*

4. Move down to the legs, and give effleurage strokes over the whole leg before moving on to petrissage, or kneading, over the thighs. Treat the thigh as three sections, outer, middle and inner, and knead up and down each section. Massage of the inner thigh can be quite useful during labour. The benefits are increased if the woman practises letting go all her muscles towards the massaging hands, including the muscles of the pelvic floor.

5. Another movement which works on the inner thigh is to place your open palms on either side of the thigh. Press them together, slide them up the thigh a little, repeat the pressure, slide them up and so on, till you reach the top of the thigh. Repeat on the other thigh, the woman continuing to relax her muscles towards your hands. Follow with effleurage over the whole leg. *(Overleaf top)*

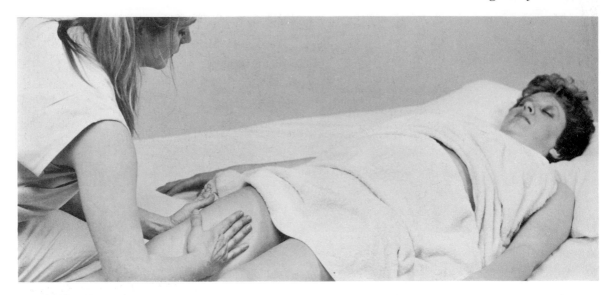

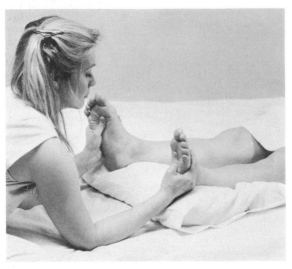

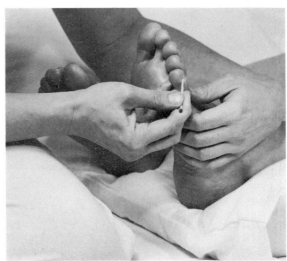

**6.** Feet are particularly responsive to mass-age during pregnancy. I have noticed that the baby usually becomes very active as the mother's feet are massaged! Stroke the top of the foot, then clasp your hands over the instep and work on the sole with your thumbs. Stroke and rotate each toe in turn.

**7.** Some women have found that it helps, during labour, to have their feet held firmly with pressure on the instep. Stand or kneel at the woman's feet and hold them with your thumbs pressing into the central hollow under the ball of the foot. Since this point relates to the diaphragm in reflexology, it is possible that this relaxes the breathing. *(Bottom left)*

**8.** There is a pressure point on the outside of the nail of the little toe which is used in the East to ease delivery. Only use it from the time

the baby is due. Press the point with a matchstick or toothpick, hard enough to feel it, but not hard enough to hurt, for a second or two, three or four times a day. *(Bottom right)*

## Massage after birth

In parts of the East women are massaged every day for three weeks after giving birth, to help the abdomen regain its tone and to allow the womb to move back into position more quickly. After each massage the abdomen is bound with long strips of cloth for support. Here are some massage strokes which may help the mother get back into shape.

**1.** Begin with the two kinds of effleurage shown on pages 28 and 29, that is the continu-

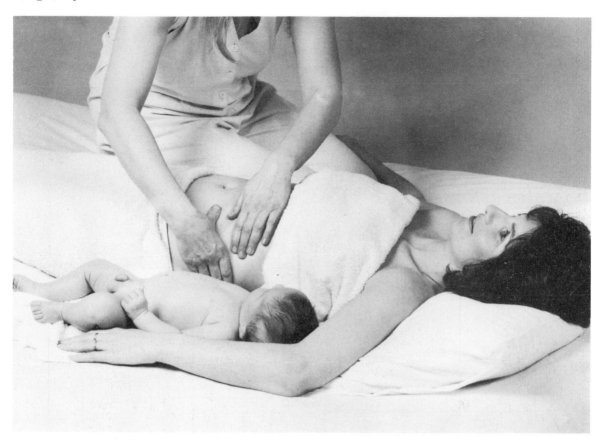

ous circular effleurage and straight effleurage up over the ribs, round the back and down towards the groin.

**2.** Petrissage or kneading helps to tone the muscles and break up fatty tissue. Do not knead directly over the womb, but concentrate your attention around the sides of the body, particularly the top of the hips and the waist-line. *(Above)*

**3.** If the mother has any stretch-marks, they can be reduced by 'miniature petrissage', an alternating rolling pinch between thumbs and forefingers across the grain of each stretch-mark. Do this gently but persistently, working only on the surface of the tissues.

**4.** This is a stroke Indian midwives use: one long, slow, deep stroke from the pubic bone to the breastbone. If it is done correctly, with a relaxed hand, your hand should make a sucking noise as it comes off the chest at the top of the stroke. The mother may feel her abdominal muscles contract as your hand strokes upward. *(Right)* Do this stroke four or five times, and finish with the two methods of effleurage.

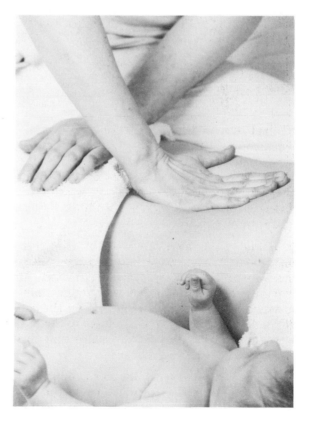

# BABIES AND CHILDREN

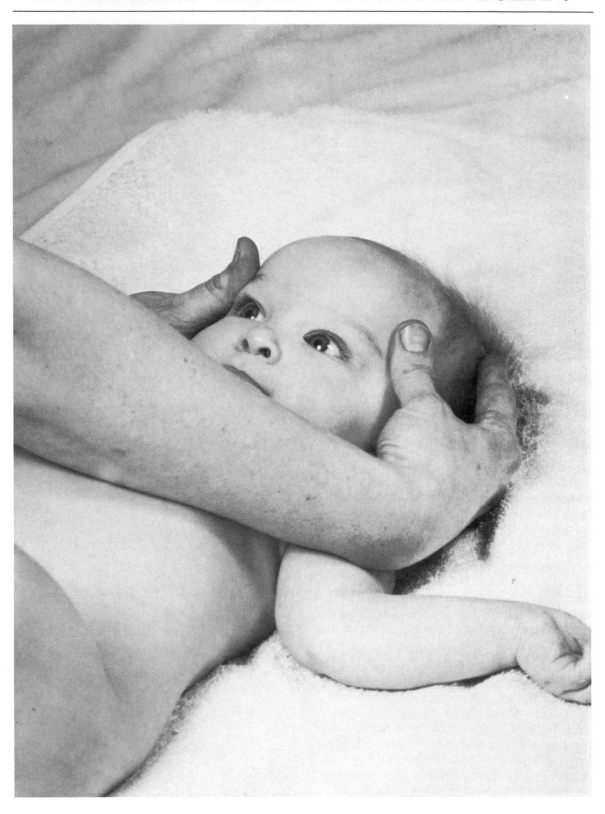

# Babies

Birth is a trauma in itself, and difficult births are more traumatic for both mother and baby. Gentle massaging of your baby can help make up for this difficult start. In South American clinics specializing in premature births, babies who look like giving up the fight are tempted back to life by a drop or two of fruit juice on the tongue and a massage! Massage can also help build up the mother's confidence in handling her baby, and for the baby, it is an introduction to loving touch which can encourage him, or her, to feel secure and trusting in the world. It is a good idea for the father to take an occasional turn at massaging his baby, as fathers so often miss out on physical contact.

Round about bath-time in the evening, and not too close to a feed, is a good time to massage your baby; try to make it a part of the regular routine. The room, your hands, and the oil, should be warm, and remember to take off rings and bracelets. Lay the baby on a nappy and have a flannel handy in case of accidents. You can use oil, lotion or powder on your baby, but essences may be too strong for a baby's delicate skin.

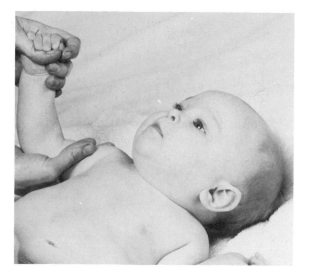

1. Begin with the face – do not use any oil here – to capture your baby's attention and establish eye contact. Keep eye contact with your baby throughout the massage, and talk to her as well. Cradle the baby's head in your hands and stroke outwards with your thumbs over the forehead, from the nose out over the cheeks, and from the chin up to the ears. Do each stroke a couple of times, then stroke downwards on either side of the ears, with thumbs one side, fingers the other, and with your fingers carry on down the sides of the neck to the shoulders. *(Opposite)*

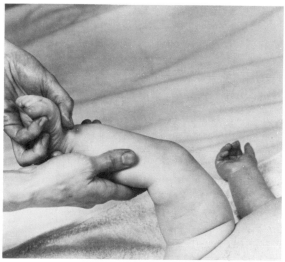

2. Now oil first your hands, then the baby. Spread the oil from the chest out over the arms, then from the tummy down over the legs. Now work on each arm at a time; hold the arm up with one hand, and with the other work from wrist to shoulder with little rhythmic, moving, squeezing movements. *(Top)* Make circles on the front and back of the hand with your thumb and forefinger, and stroke each finger in turn.

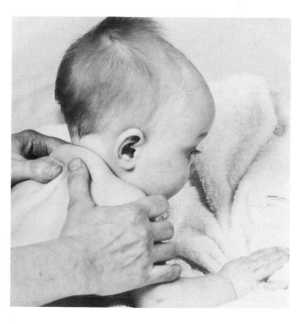

3. Stroke the baby's chest from the centre outwards, moving down to the tummy. Make

continuous circular stroking movements on the tummy, with one hand following the other.

**4.** Work on the legs as on the arms, holding each leg up in turn. Finish by massaging each foot with your thumb on the sole, and pulling the toes gently. *(Previous page middle right)*

**5.** Stroke the entire front of the baby's body a few times, right down to the feet. Now turn the baby on to her front.

**6.** With your hands resting on the baby's shoulders, move your thumbs in tiny circles down the back of the neck and increase the size of the circles as you reach the area between the shoulder blades. Keep the circular movement going as you go down the back, so that your thumbs are massaging the whole back area, while your fingers are gently holding her sides and tummy. *(Previous page bottom right)*

**7.** Finish with long, gentle strokes all the way down the back, starting with your palm, and getting lighter and lighter until you are barely touching with your fingertips.

# Children

If children are massaged from birth (and you can start from the first week) they will grow up familiar with the caring touch and will happily massage their parents. Their concentration does not last long, however, so it is a good idea to make the massage session as much of a game as possible. One of the games which is most fun for both them and you is the game of 'Walking on Grown-ups' Backs'. A child of under ten walking up and down your back provides just the right amount of pressure to ease aching muscles, and even if the child overbalances, the teetering little feet can feel delicious!

As for massaging children themselves, they take to it very quickly, and love it. It is good for them, too and children respond much more quickly to massage therapy than adults, because their systems are more sensitive. Many of my students, practising on their children, have reported that temper tantrums have ceased, hyperactivity has disappeared, and infantile eczema has shown an improvement. In the Far East, massage is used as a matter of course, not just to strengthen the child's constitution but also to treat minor ailments. Here are two strokes from China that you might like to incorporate into your massage.

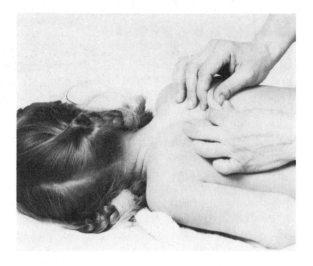

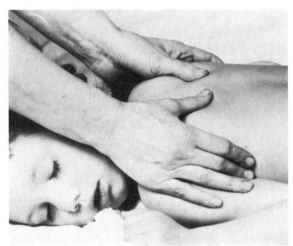

**1.** *'Pinch-pull' movement.* This stroke can be used from babyhood onward to strengthen a child's digestive system. Take a pinch of flesh between your thumbs and forefingers at the base of the child's spine on one side, and roll it upwards with your thumbs. Take up the same position of fingers and thumbs a half-inch or so further up the back and repeat, and so on all the way up the back. The effect of the movement is that you are moving the flesh upwards, away from the bone, in a long strip next to the spine. Repeat on the other side. *(Top)*

**2.** *Circling the shoulders.* This movement is used in China to strengthen a child's lungs, if he, or she, has a tendency to be 'chesty'. Resting your hands on the top of the child's shoulders, sweep your thumbs down around the shoulder blades, from top to bottom and out to the sides. Repeat this movement at least twenty times a day, every day, to strengthen the chest. *(Bottom)*

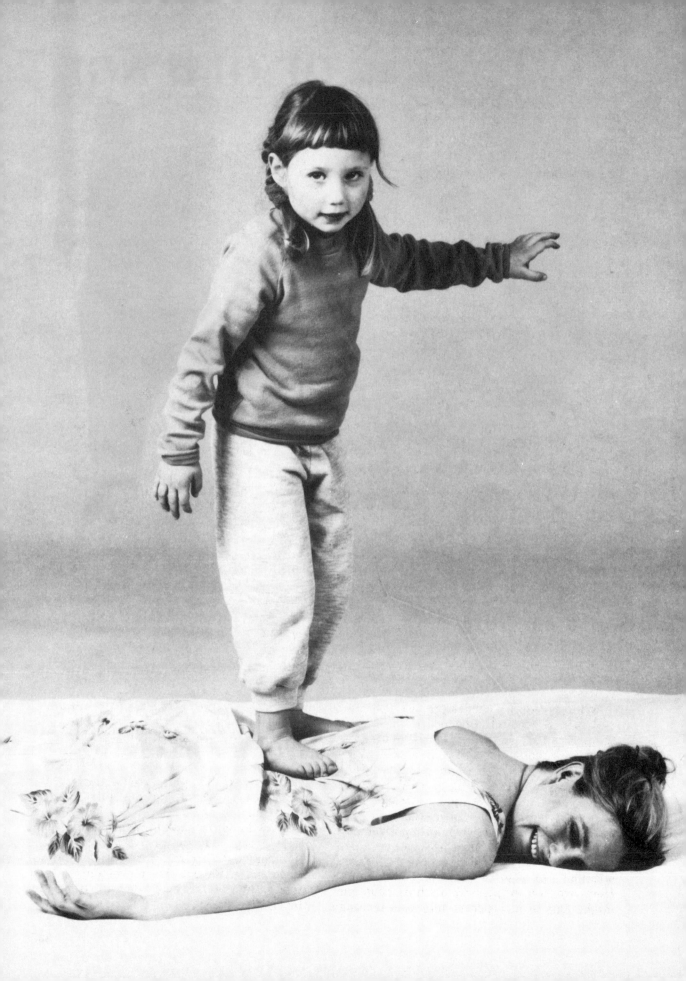

# PROBLEMS OF OLD AGE

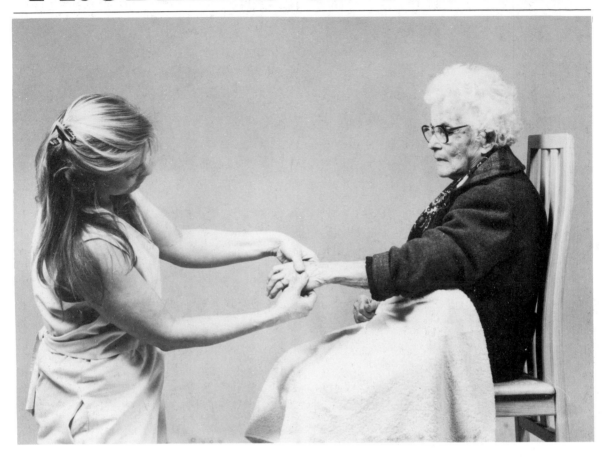

With a healthy diet, adequate rest and exercise and above all a positive, vital approach to life, old age can be a serene and fulfilling time. However, it's also a time when wear and tear takes its toll, usually on the muscles and joints, resulting in aches and pains which are often labelled 'arthritis'. In fact, many of these aches can be relieved by massage as well as by drugs, especially if the massage is done with herbal essences.

## Oils for arthritis and rheumatism

Always remember to dilute your essences in a carrier oil, although for this purpose you can use slightly higher concentrations than previously – about eight drops of essence to half a teacupful of carrier oil. If the condition feels worse in cold weather, use warming essences such as rosemary or marjoram; if it feels worse in heat, think of cooling ones such as peppermint or camomile. Lavender should always be included, as it is a good pain-reliever, and I usually add juniper, as a de-toxifier.

A word of warning; *if an arthritic joint is inflamed, that is, it feels hot to the touch and is red, do not massage it.* Instead you can apply a herbal compress, and massage the surrounding areas to relax the muscles and improve the lymph drainage.

## Arthritic hands

Pain in the hands is a common problem as we get older. This hand massage will help relieve stiffness and pain.
**1.** As you oil the hand, spread it open with a slow movement outwards of your thumbs on the front of the hand. Keep your fingers on the back of the hand. *(Above)*

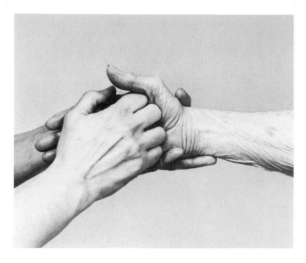

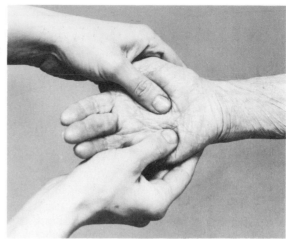

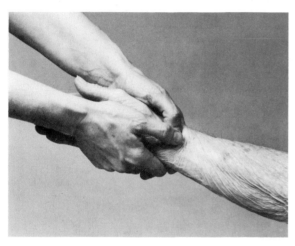

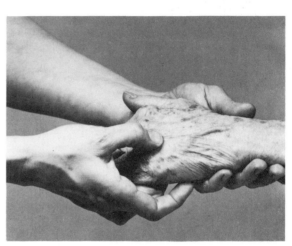

**2.** Support the hand palm upwards with one of your own. With the other, in a loose fist, make circular movements with your knuckle in the palm. *(Top left)*

**3.** Supporting the hand, still palm upwards, with the fingers of both your hands, use your thumbs to make tiny circles in the palm, covering the whole surface. *(Top right)*

**4.** Still supporting the hand with your fingers, make tiny circular movements with your thumbs down the wrist, from where the thumb ends at the wrist joint. Sometimes what passes for arthritis can be friction between the tendon and its sheath at this point. This movement can really relieve pain in the thumbs. *(Middle left)*

**5.** Turn the hand over and support it at the wrist with one hand. With the other hand, thumb above, index finger below, drain between the bones of the hand out to the web between the fingers. *(Middle right)*

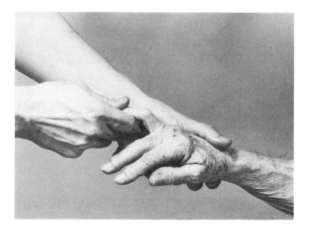

**6.** Pull each finger in turn – pull along the sides of the fingers, as they are more sensitive – pump each joint and rotate each finger. *(Bottom right)*

**7.** To finish, enclose the hand in both your own and draw them both very slowly along it and off the ends of the fingers.

# Back problems

Elderly people may find it hard to lie face down for a back massage, especially if you work on the floor. So why not massage them while they are sitting astride the back of a chair, as we showed on page 26. You can use any of the strokes suggested there, but you might like to try these extra strokes, especially good for the stiff backs and necks of the elderly.

**1.** Starting at the base of the spine, slide your thumbs slowly and deeply up the muscles on each side of the spinal column and along the top of the shoulders when you get to the top. You can vary this movement by applying rhythmic pressure with your thumbs as you slide them up, and also by continuing up the back of the neck instead of out along the shoulders. Keep the rest of your hand in contact with the back. *(Top right)*

**2.** Make tiny, deep circular movements along the base of the skull with both thumbs, moving from the centre out towards the ears. You may want to support your friend's head with your fingers on the temples, for extra steadiness, or simply leave the head tilted forwards. *(Bottom right)*

# Knee problems

The knee is a major weight-bearing joint, and is thus liable to deterioration as time goes on. As the joint builds up extra bone to protect itself, it swells, and all the surrounding muscles tense up to stabilize the painful knee. Massage for this condition aims to improve the circulation and remove extra fluid from the knee joint, and also to ease the pain in the surrounding muscles.

For many older people, the sitting position is the most comfortable one in which to receive massage. The giver can sit either in a chair, which involves a certain amount of bending, or sit on the floor.

**1.** After oiling the leg, stroke up it from ankle to knee, with your thumbs crossed over the shin and your hands moulded around the sides of the calf. As you come to the knee, give a little squeeze with your fingers around the back of it, then bring your hands around and slide the flat of both hands gently down the shin to the ankle. Repeat. *(Opposite top)*

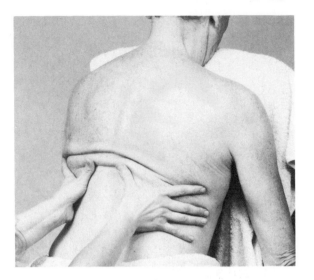

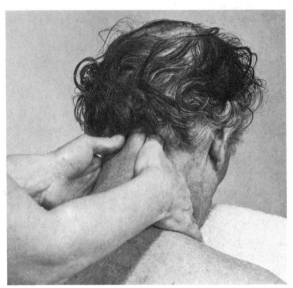

**2.** With your thumbs overlapping just below the knee cap and your fingers resting on the sides of the knee, circle the knee cap with your thumbs.

**3.** With your hands in the same starting position, do little circular frictions with your thumbs all around the edges of the knee cap.

**4.** With alternating hands, stroke firmly up the back of the knee with a diagonal movement, moulding your hands to the contours of the leg. *(Opposite bottom left)*

# Reflexology

Foot massage is one of the most ancient healing arts, rediscovered in this century and

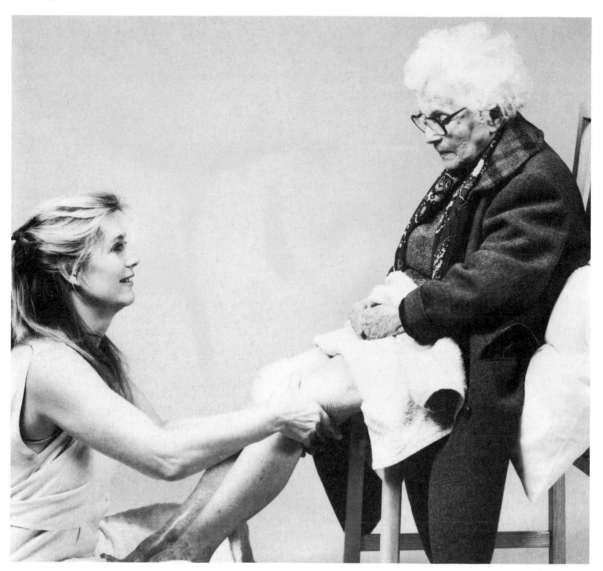

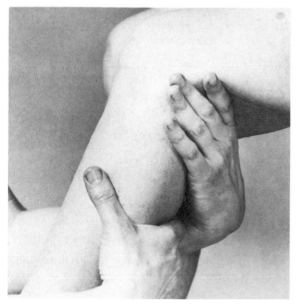

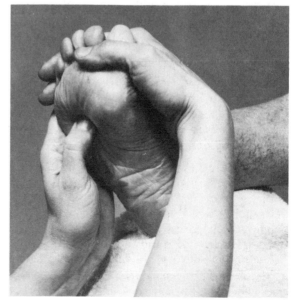

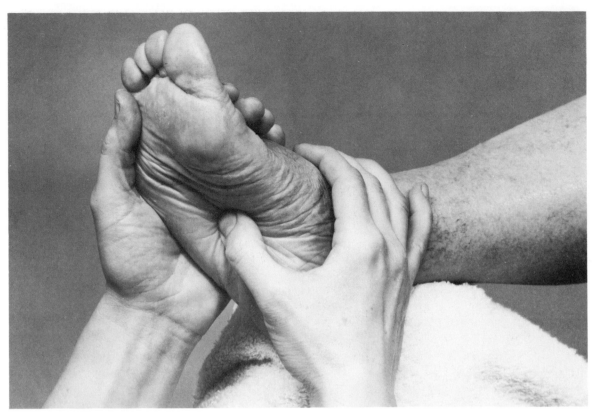

named reflexology. It works on the theory that the feet are a map of the body, with reflex points relating to each organ or body structure; thus through treating the feet we can indirectly treat the whole body. Reflexology is a wonderful treatment for older people, who might at first feel reluctant to undress for a full body massage. There are many good books on this fascinating subject, but here I will give you an idea of a sample treatment to help an arthritic knee, which you can incorporate into the leg massage routine given above, while the foot is on your lap. Do not oil the foot.

**1.** Stroke the *right* foot several times, toes to ankle, top and bottom.

**2.** Hold your partner's foot at the toes to support it, and with your thumb press along the area on the outside of the instep, just under the ball of the foot. Press repeatedly, moving your thumb at tiny intervals to cover the area, which is more or less a square inch. This is the liver and gallbladder reflex (on the right foot only, as these organs are located on the right-hand side of the body) and may be useful in detoxifying the system. (*Previous page bottom right*)

**3.** Move your thumb down to a spot in the very centre of the instep, which is the kidney reflex. (*Above*) Often the reflex points are detectable by their tenderness to the touch, or you may feel a slightly 'crunchy' sensation under your thumb, which can indicate deposits or congestion in the organ concerned. Stroke with your thumb from the kidney reflex down towards the bladder reflex, which is on the lower edge of the instep, where it joins the heel. This movement is said to help waste products eliminated from the kidneys to pass down the ureters to the bladder for disposal. Since arthritis is often connected with poor elimination of waste products from the system, this stimulation of the kidneys may well be helpful. (*Opposite top*)

**4.** The foot reflex area for the knee itself is on the outside edge of the foot, next to the heel and below the ankle. Work on this with your thumb or fingers, 'walking' along the area with rhythmic pressures. The reflex will probably be more painful on the side where the knee gives most trouble. Both this movement and the kidney-bladder stimulation shown above can be done on both feet. (*Opposite bottom*)

**5.** Finish by stroking the whole foot once again.

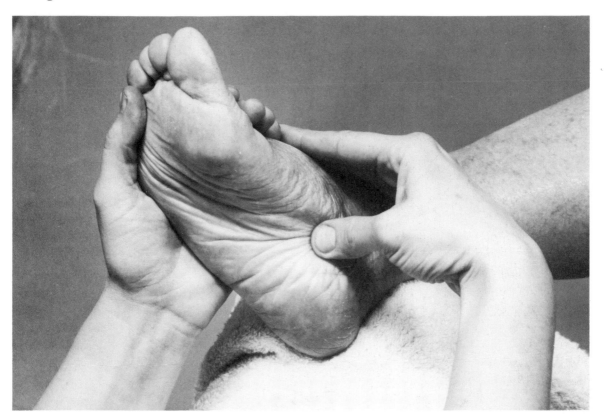

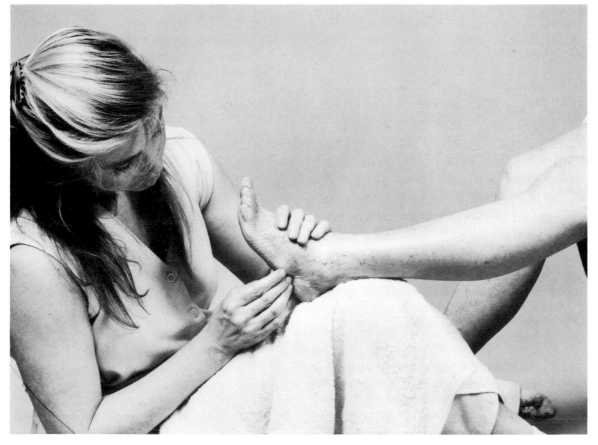

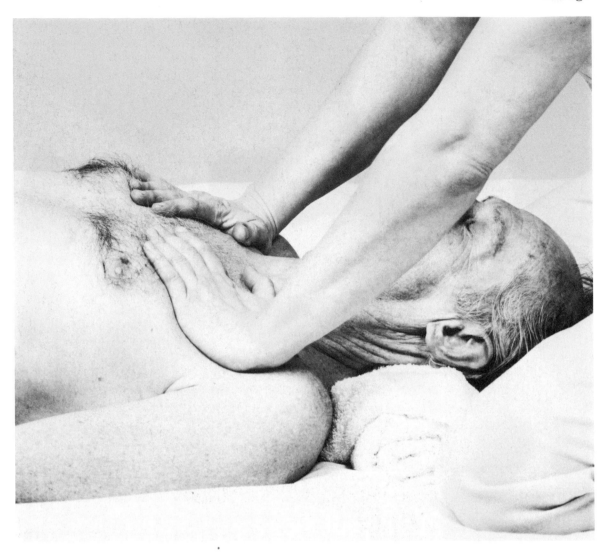

# Massage for heart problems

Heart disease is a rapidly growing problem in this country, and the experts associate it not only with smoking, saturated fats in the diet and lack of exercise, but also with stress. We all suffer from stress, of course, but for the type of person prone to heart disease, much of the stress is self-inflicted. This type of personality (often referred to as Type 'A', to distinguish him from the relaxed, easy-going Type 'B') is active, energetic and tries hard, sometimes too hard. Obviously, relaxation is indicated (although the Type 'A' person will avoid this strenuously!) and massage can be a valuable aid to relaxation, thus possibly helping to pre-

vent heart disease. If heart disease *does* strike, however, gentle massage can do a great deal to eliminate the discomfort and depression which follow a heart attack. Massage is currently being tried at a major London teaching hospital as a recovery aid for cardiac patients, and the results have been good. Obviously there are cases when massage is not advisable, *so do consult a doctor first.*

1. To relax the shoulders and chest, sit behind your partner as he lies on his back. Oil the chest with long, smooth strokes. Then stroke outward and downward with both hands from just below the throat, fanning your hands out across the chest and around the arms *(Above)*; then bring your hands up under the shoulders and up the back of the neck. This is an effleurage movement, so keep your pressure light on the chest; when working under the

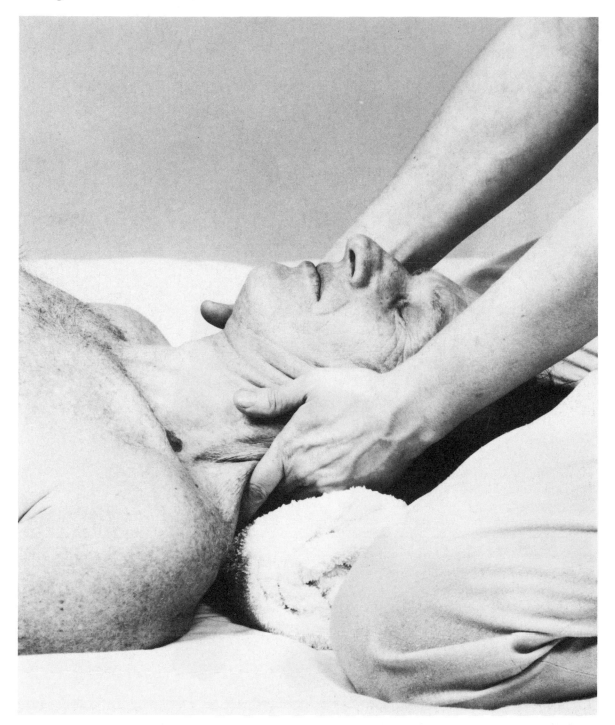

shoulders, you can allow your partner's weight to contribute to the depth of the stroke. After repeating the movement once or twice, vary it by adding a rotary movement of your fingers at the back of the neck to relax the muscles. *(Above)*

**2.** Sometimes heart problems are accompanied by an increase of fluid in the legs and ankles, which massage can help to relieve. Give gentle effleurage upwards, with your hands moulded to the front of the leg, and then draw them lightly back down the sides.

**3.** The heart reflex lies on the centre of the ball of the left foot, but your partner may feel a bit lopsided if you do not treat both feet. 'Walk' your thumb gently across the ball of the foot.

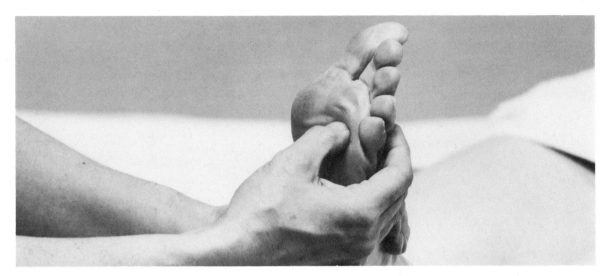

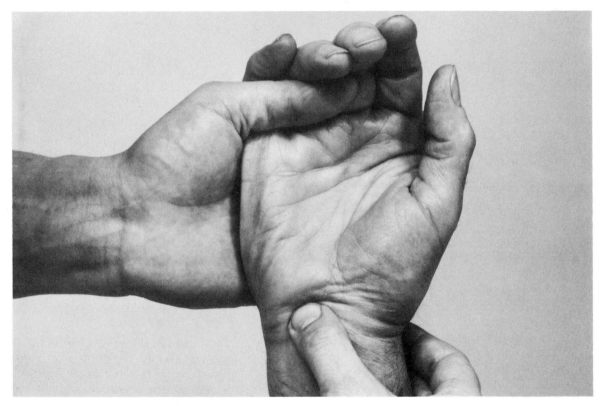

Do not overwork the heart reflex. *(Top)* Follow with a general massage of the sole of the foot with the heel of your hand, supporting the top of the foot with your other palm.

**4.** Gentle effleurage up the arms will also help the circulation and after doing this you can press an acupuncture point which not only benefits the heart but can help relieve the anxiety and depression which so often accompanies heart problems. The point is on the wrist crease, under the bone on the little finger side. Bend the wrist so that you can angle your thumb in, and move your thumb around a little until you find the right spot; your partner can usually feel it. Press gently for two seconds, three or four times. *(Bottom)*

**5.** Pulling the little finger (especially the left one) is an acupressure treatment for the heart. Pull along the sides of the finger, and press firmly on the sides of the nail as you slide off.

# ATHLETES

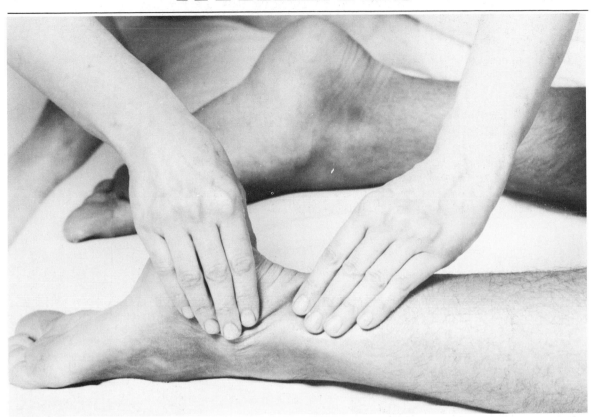

Over the last few years there has been an enormous increase of interest in fitness and exercise; our parks are filled with joggers, our church halls with aerobic dance classes. And sports injuries are on the increase too, leading to dire warnings from the experts that exercise can be bad for you. What is not generally known is that massage can be a superb aid to the athlete. Most professional athletes are massaged several times a week to keep their muscles in good condition and minimize the possibilities of injury; but for slightly less intensive exercisers once a week or once a fortnight will do.

When training, muscles become shorter; and they often shorten unevenly, so that posture imbalances develop. This is when injury becomes a real possibility. Massage lengthens and relaxes the muscles and irons out unevenness, so that injuries can be avoided. It can also help when an old injury impairs the effectiveness of a muscle or joint. For most forms of exercise, running, jumping, dancing and so on, massage of the legs and back will be sufficient

(although a full body massage is more relaxing). I have already covered the back in some detail, *(see page 11)* so here is a leg massage for sports fanatics.

## Leg massage

### The back of the legs

**1.** Begin by oiling the leg, followed directly by effleurage. This should be a long firm slow stroke upward, with hands moulded around the leg, increasing the pressure slightly over the thigh. Slide the hands gently down the sides of the leg and off the foot. Then stroke firmly up the leg again (without pressing too hard over the knee). This firm stroking helps to lengthen the muscle fibres.

**2.** Petrissage is one of the mose useful movements for increasing circulation to the muscles. Begin at the back of the ankle, grasping the Achilles tendon between thumb and fingers with small but deep kneading movements. *(Above)* Move your kneading hands up over

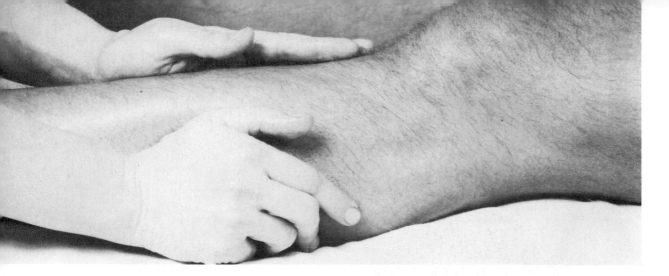

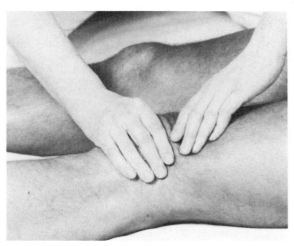

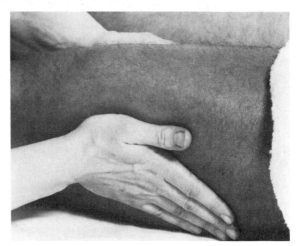

the calf muscle, taking the muscle up with a larger area of the hand.

**3.** Moving up to the thigh, treat it as three sections, inner, middle and outer. Knead up and down each section with firm, regular movements, grasping as much of the flesh of the thigh in your hands as you can each time.

**6.** Place your hands on either side of the thigh, just above the knee and press inwards. Slide your hands a little further up and press inwards again. Continue up to the top of the thigh, then return to the beginning and repeat the sequence. The muscles of the side of the thigh are important in maintaining balance, and therefore affect the knee and hip joints.

### The front of the legs

**1.** Oil the front of the leg. Give effleurage over the whole limb, moulding your hands, as always, to the contours of the leg, and allowing them to flow smoothly over the knee cap. As

you draw your hands gently down the leg, include the foot as you slide off.

**2.** The shin consists of half bone and half muscle, so you treat it with a half-and-half movement. Slide one hand slowly up the bony side in an effleurage movement, while the other hand moves up at the same pace on the muscular side, making deep rotary movements with the heel of the hand. When you reach the knee, draw the hands lightly down the sides of the leg and repeat the sequence. *(Top)*

**3.** Facing your partner's leg, grasp the knee cap with alternate hands as if you were doing petrissage. Grasp the sides of the knee cap between thumb and fingers, slide along the knee, then release. Immediately grasp the knee with the other hand, slide it in the other direction, then release. *(Bottom left)*

**4.** For the front of the thigh, divide it into three sections as for the back, and give petrissage. Follow with the press-slide movement on

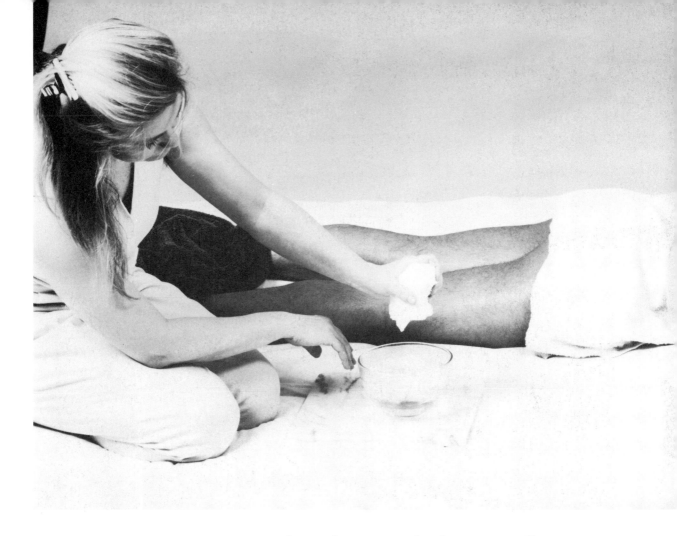

the sides of the thigh, *(Opposite right)* exactly as when working on the back of the leg, and finish with effleurage over the whole leg.

# Remedial massage for injuries

If you are new to exercise, do bear in mind that Massage is a terrific way of improving performance, as well as preventing injuries. Obviously, you need to pay attention to other common-sense measures as well, such as warm clothing (muscles tear when cold), proper sports shoes, and of course a well-balanced diet. Do remember to do warm-ups before launching into strenuous exercise; sustained stretches lengthen the muscle fibres, rather than 'bouncing' stretches, which actually shorten them.

If for some reason you do injure yourself while exercising, the best first-aid treatment is rest, combined with cold compresses, for at least twenty-four hours, or until the area is no longer tender to the touch. Applying a cold compress is a simple procedure. Fill a quart-sized bowl with cold water and ice. Dip a cloth such as a muslin nappy or a small towel in the water, wring it out slightly and apply it to the injured area. Hold it there for a few seconds, then dip the cloth in the water again and repeat the process as often as possible. *(Above)* This reduces internal bleeding in the muscle and inflammation. After the compress you could apply a little lavender or camomile essence diluted in oil, to aid healing. After the pain subsides, a little gentle effleurage over the area can be the start of remedial massage treatment – but do not start this till the muscle has had a chance to heal.

If an old injury is causing trouble, massage can sometimes clear up the trouble completely, or at least maintain the problem limb in good enough condition to continue exercising.

**1.** The remedial technique used by Guy Og-

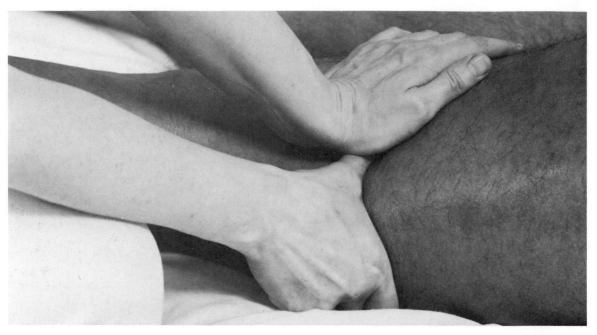

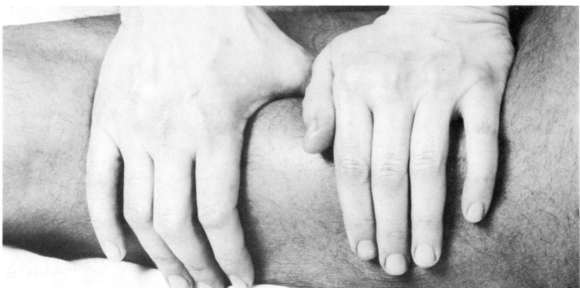

den, the osteopath featured in our programme on sports injuries, is a very slow, deep stroke along the grain of the muscle, using one hand over the thumb of the other for extra pressure. As muscle tears heal in a lumpy fashion, this movement helps to separate the clumped muscle fibres and clear away any waste products around an old injury. *(Top)*

**2.** After several minutes of this deep length-wise stroking, or when the muscle feels softer and less lumpy, do a few similar movements *across* the grain of the muscle, at right angles to your previous movements. *(Bottom)*

Remember that each muscle works in conjunction with other muscles as part of a whole, so try to include your remedial massage for old injuries in a general massage, if not of the whole body then at least of the whole area. For example, if the injured area is a hamstring, massage both legs thoroughly as well as using your remedial technique on the injured area.

# Hot & cold compresses

You learnt on page 47 how to treat a recent

injury with cold compresses. When the injury has had a little time to heal, or in the case of an old injury which has been neglected, alternate hot and cold compresses can be very helpful. You will need two quart-sized bowls, one filled with cold water and ice, the other one with water as hot as your hand can comfortably take, and two cloths. Squeeze out a cloth in the hot water, apply it to the injured area with quite firm pressure and wait half a minute or so. Do the same with the cold water over the same spot – your friend will probably yelp! – then repeat with the hot water. *(Above right)* Continue alternating the compresses for five or six changes, finishing with a cold one. The area should go pink, showing an increase in the local circulation. At a pinch, you could use a bathroom spray over the painful area, alternating hot and cold water, finishing with cold, but a heating pad is not the answer – dry heat is not as effective as wet heat.

As a massage oil for injured muscles, when the injury is chronic rather than acute, add rosemary or marjoram to your lavender and camomile mixture, to increase the circulation. And as a general muscle-toner, lemongrass is said to be beneficial, and many athletes use it to keep their muscles in good condition.

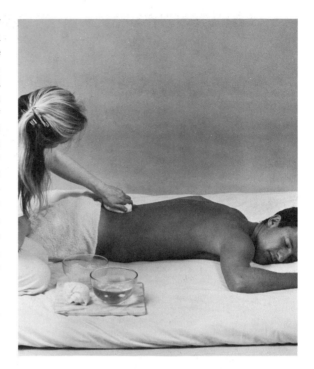

# Massage for back pain

Even if you do not exercise, this remedial technique can be of value in treating muscular aches and pains, such as lower back pain. In very many cases, back pain comes from the muscles and ligaments rather than from displaced vertebrae or intervertebral discs. So, if the cause of your pain is muscular, the same measures apply as for sports injuries; if the problem is acute, rest and cold compresses, if the problem is long-standing or chronic, remedial massage, with hot *and* cold compresses.

**1.** Work on the fibrous, knotted muscle in the back with the same deep, slow, penetrating stroking movement as demonstrated above. You can work with both thumbs or with one thumb and the other hand on top of it to achieve the right depth of pressure.

**2.** The muscles of the hips, just below the waist on both sides, are often involved in lower back pain. Even if the pain is felt elsewhere, these muscles are often tight and knotted, so do deep stroking upwards along these muscles, too. Do not try and work on both hips from the same

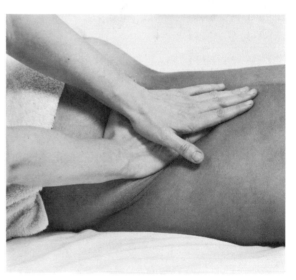

side – change your position for extra leverage. *(Below right)*

**3.** Remember that to function normally the back muscles need to work together in harmony; the key is *balance*. So work on both sides of the back with effleurage and all the other strokes demonstrated in the first chapter, so that the back feels like a whole, and all the muscles are free to work with each other.

**4.** You can also use hot and cold compresses for back pain, as described in the section on chronic injury treatment.

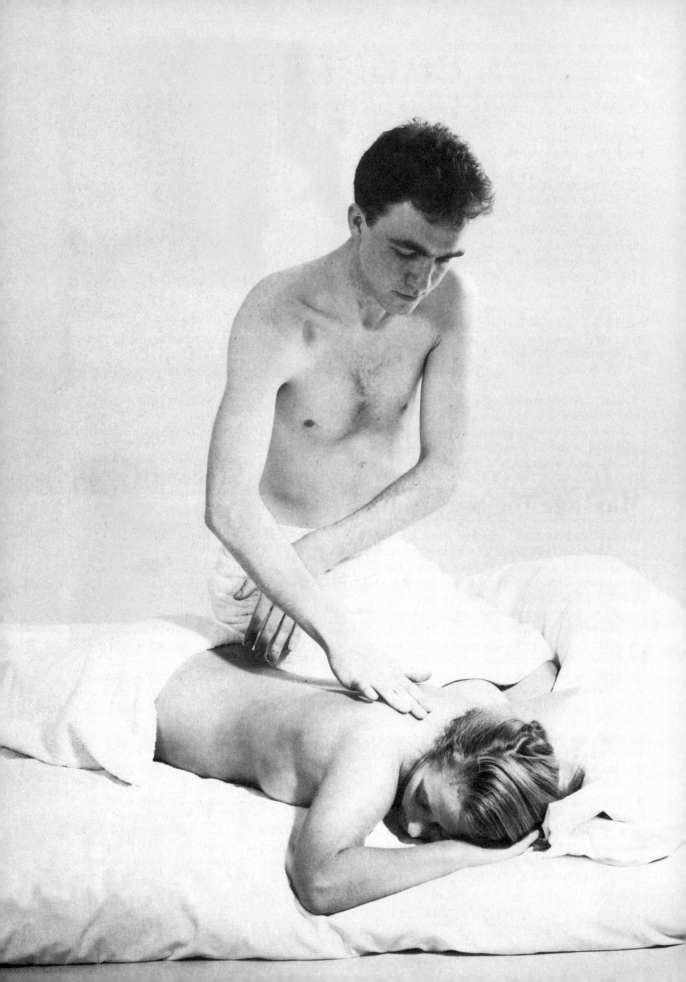

# COUPLES

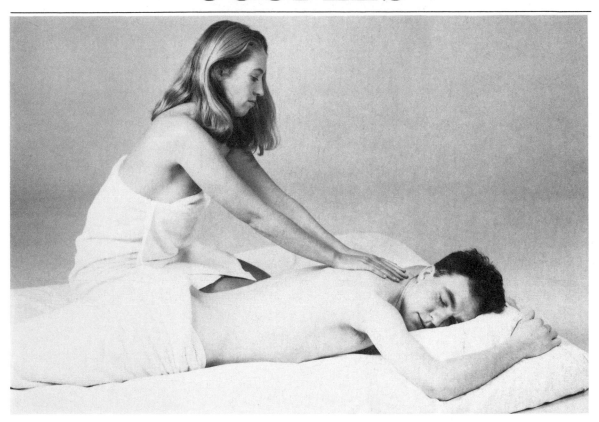

Up until now, we have been seeing how massage can heal and relax where there is pain, tension or discomfort. Now let us look at massage as a form of loving communication. There is nothing as reassuring as touch; it takes us back to the protective bond between mother and baby, the physical contact which meant love, security and trust. As we grow older, so we grow away from this natural contact and forget how to communicate affection through touch. But we can re-learn it through massage, and nowhere is massage more appropriate than in the couple situation. In the helter-skelter of twentieth-century life almost everyone is overstressed, and marriages or partnerships easily lose the first flush of love and intimacy as the demands of the outside world take their toll. It is really worth taking time off together in peace and quiet to give each other a massage. It is a new way of relating to your partner's body – playful, gentle and undemanding. Try it, and see how much closer you feel. You can use any of the strokes in the rest of the book, or try the suggestions here.

## The back of the body

### The back and shoulders

1. Learn the shape of your partner's body with your hands. The most loving stroke is slow effleurage, with all your attention focused in your hands as they slide very slowly upwards and return gently down the sides of the back. With this slow, rhythmic movement you will soon find that you are in harmony with your partner's energies, and your hands will detect areas of tension and know how to soothe them away. *(Above)*

You may want to stay with the stroking movement, making it lighter or deeper, quicker or slower as the mood takes you; or you may feel like going into a full back routine as in Chapter I *(see page 11)*; kneading up one side of the back, across the shoulders, up the neck and down the other side of the back; circular frictions up the sides of the spine and down the edges of the shoulder-blades. I personally do

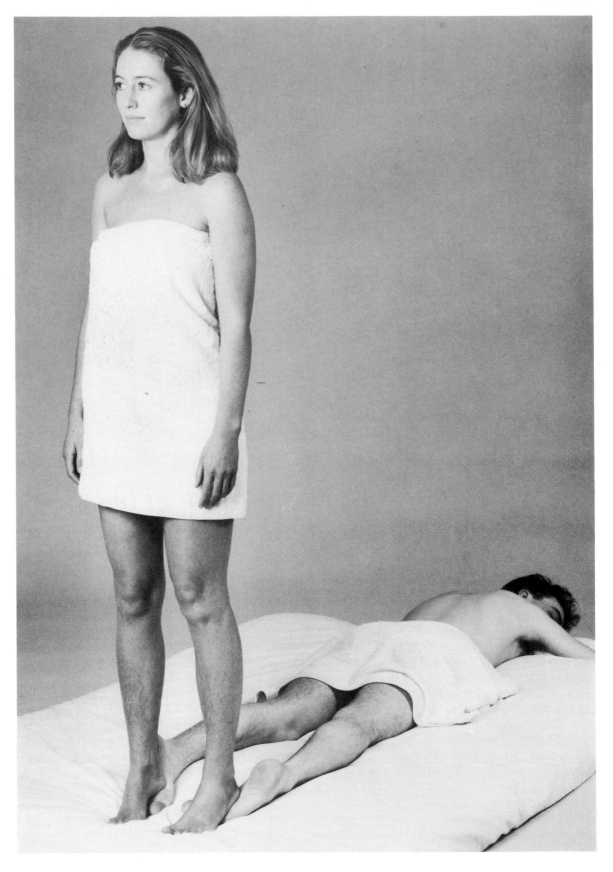

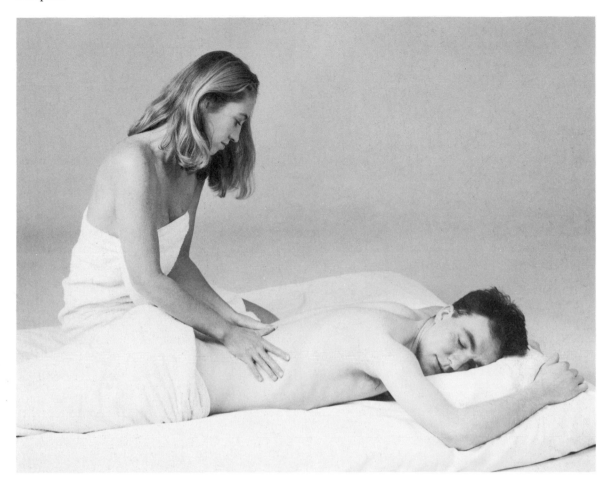

not think that percussion movements would be right in this context. They are stimulating rather than relaxing, and certainly not a good idea if there is any hidden tension between you and your partner! You can include the buttocks in all these back strokes – massage here can be very relaxing, especially for women.

**2.** Feather-light stroking to finish is a lovely movement to do for someone you love. Stroke down the back from top to bottom with your fingertips, very light and feathery, with your hands following each other in sequence. The gentleness of this movement can be very relaxing. *(Page 50)*

### The backs of the legs

Now you can work on the backs of the legs, with effleurage, petrissage (knead the thigh in three sections, as it is a larger area) and the press-and-slide movement on the sides of the thigh – check the Legs sequence on page 16. You can go right up on to the hip and buttock area on your partner (here is one occasion when you do not have to feel shy) to make the limb feel connected to the body.

If your partner is on the floor, try walking on his or her feet before turning him or her over.

# The front of the body

### The face

Massage of the face can be the most delicious experience, as all problems are literally stroked away. Sit behind your partner's head for this sequence. Spread a little oil on your hands first and stroke it lightly over the skin before beginning to massage.

**1.** Stroke with relaxed palms out from the centre of the face to the sides, from the chin out over the jaw, and from the nose out over the cheeks to the ears. *(Overleaf top left)*

**2.** Stroke up the forehead with a rolling movement of your fingers, one hand following smoothly upon the other, and covering the surface of the forehead. *(Overleaf top right)*

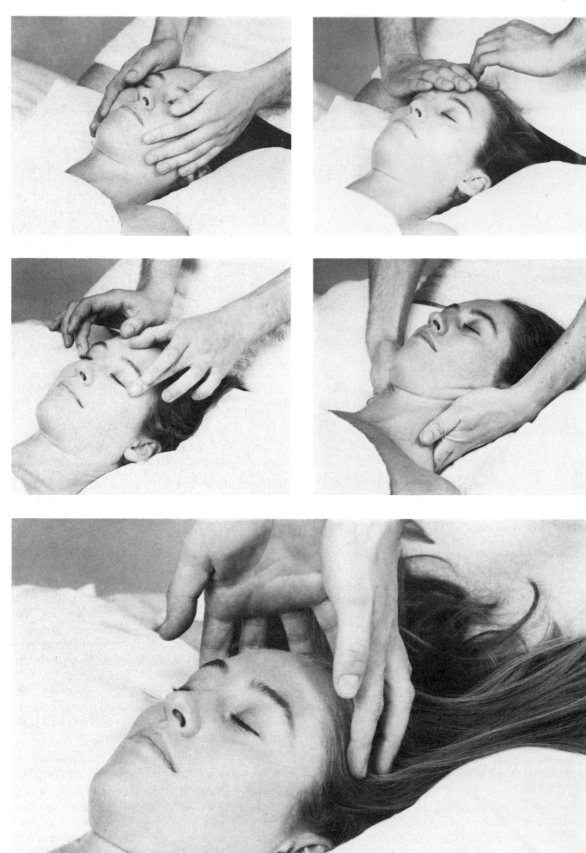

**3.** Pinch gently with thumb and forefinger out along the eyebrows, from centre to sides.

**4.** Gently circle the eyes with your middle fingers, from the inner corner around the bone of the eye socket and lightly back under the eye towards the nose. *(Opposite middle left)*

**5.** Fan your hands out across your partner's upper chest, curl them around behind the shoulders and pull them slowly, firmly, up the back of the neck and head, being careful not to pull the hair. *(Opposite middle right)*

**6.** Massage your partner's ears. Roll the ear-lobes between thumb and forefinger and then carry on the rolling movement up the rim of the ear, then down into the creases and folds.

**7.** Rake your fingers through your partner's hair, from hairline to crown. Do not be too light, since your fingers should contact the scalp. Cover the whole surface of the head in this way; if you gently turn your partner's head first to one side, then the other, you can reach the sides and back of the head too. This stroking of the scalp can be very, very pleasurable, particularly for people whose minds are always busy; it can leave them 'floating' and utterly relaxed. *(Opposite bottom)*

## The hands

Since our hands are supplied with vast numbers of sensory nerves, they are very receptive to massage. Try all the strokes on pages 36 and 37, as well as this one.

**1.** Place your little fingers under your partner's index finger and fourth finger, close to the base. Use this manoeuvre to 'open' the upturned palm. Your thumbs are then free to make circles in the palm centre. *(Right)*

**2.** Do not forget to do effleurage up your partner's arm before and after the hand massage, allowing your hands to curl around the limb so that you cover the whole arm surface, and taking your stroke right up on to the shoulder. After the final effleurage stroke, draw your hands very, very slowly down the whole length of the arm and off the hand till your fingertips lingeringly leave your partner's fingertips.

Now you can work on the belly, if you want to cover the whole of your partner's body. Follow circular effleurage on the belly by stroking up and out over the ribcage, down the sides of the back and, cresting the hipbones, back to the

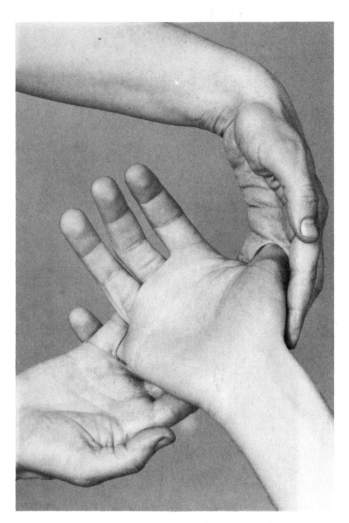

front of the body and lightly down towards the groin. Check page 28 for details.

## The front of the legs

Next, massage the front of the legs. To recap effleurage up the whole leg, half-and-half effleurage up the shin; grasping and sliding off the knee, petrissage on the thigh in three sections, press-and-slide along the sides of the thigh, followed by effleurage over the whole leg again. Next work on the feet, clasping your hands over the top of the foot while your thumbs work on the sole, massaging and rotating the toes.

Finish your massage by standing above your partner and drawing your hands very gently and slowly from the sides of the face down the sides of the neck, down the chest, ribs and belly, hips and legs and off the feet; in other words, a whole-body stroke to leave your partner feeling truly at one with his or her self.

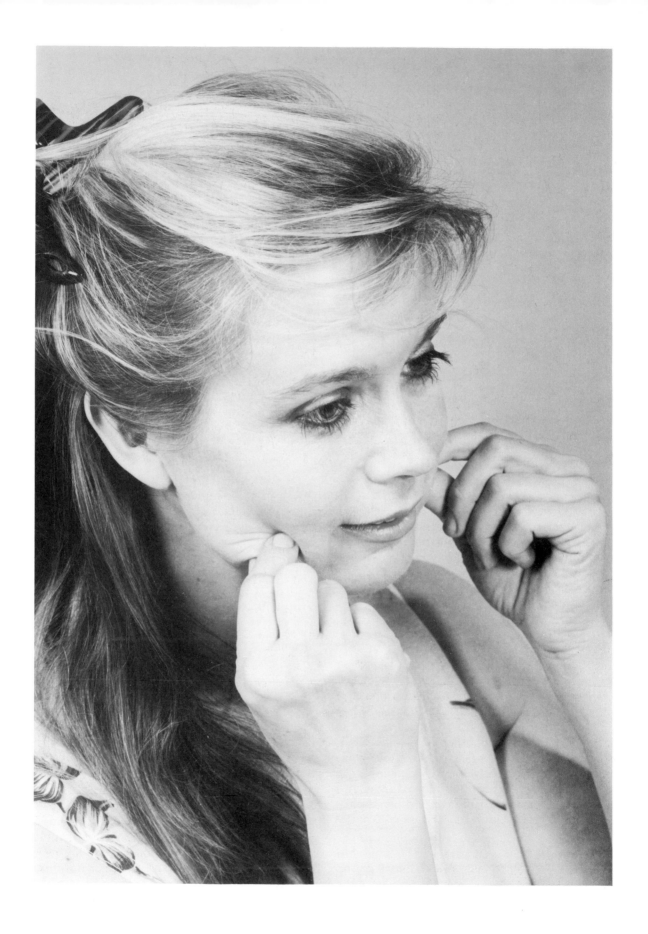

# SELF MASSAGE

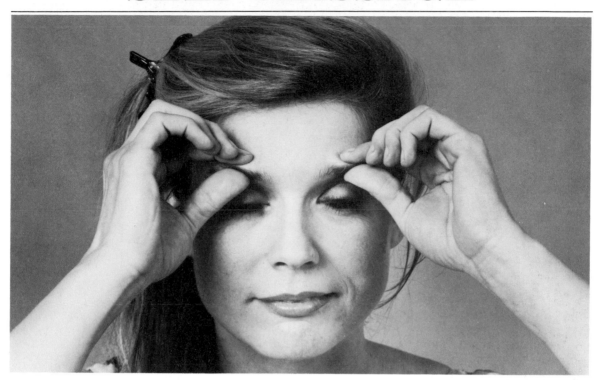

People often ask me if self massage has the same effect as being massaged by another person, and I have to say, no, it is different. Since it is you who are putting in the effort and energy, it is not a specially relaxing experience. But it *is* stimulating to the muscles, nerves and tissues, it increases the circulation and perks you up generally. Self massage also helps to put you in touch with your own body, a good thing in itself, as you learn by spending time with your body in this way to 'tune in' to its requirements, and thus increase your health, vitality and self-awareness. It is also an excellent training for massaging others, since your perception of what feels good, what pressure is painful, and so on, can help you to make others feel good, too.

You can massage yourself with or without oil, but if you use oil be careful not to use too much, as you need more grip for your hands when massaging your own body. As you will see, the techniques are different, with vigorous, stimulating movements replacing much of the stroking.

**1.** Begin with your face. Make rotary movements with your fingertips on your temples, then pinch your eyebrows between thumb and forefinger, moving from the bridge of your nose outwards. *(Above)* Circle lightly around your eyes with your middle fingers.

**2.** Make rotary movements on the jaw muscles. Pinch the jawline between your thumbs and the knuckles of your index finger, moving from your chin out towards your ears. This helps to prevent a double chin! *(Opposite)*

**3.** Massage your scalp thoroughly with your fingertips, moving the skin over the bone. Massage your ears, pulling the lobes and rolling the ears between thumb and forefinger.

**4.** Massage down the sides of your neck with big circular movements of your palms, rolling the muscles. Massage your throat more gently with rotary movements. This is helpful if you tend to get sore throats. *(Overleaf)*

**5.** Press the points at the base of your skull, halfway back from the ears, as on page 8. Roll the muscles of the back of your neck, firmly, with rotary movements; not just at the very back, but the 'sides of the back of the neck', too. *(Overleaf top left)*

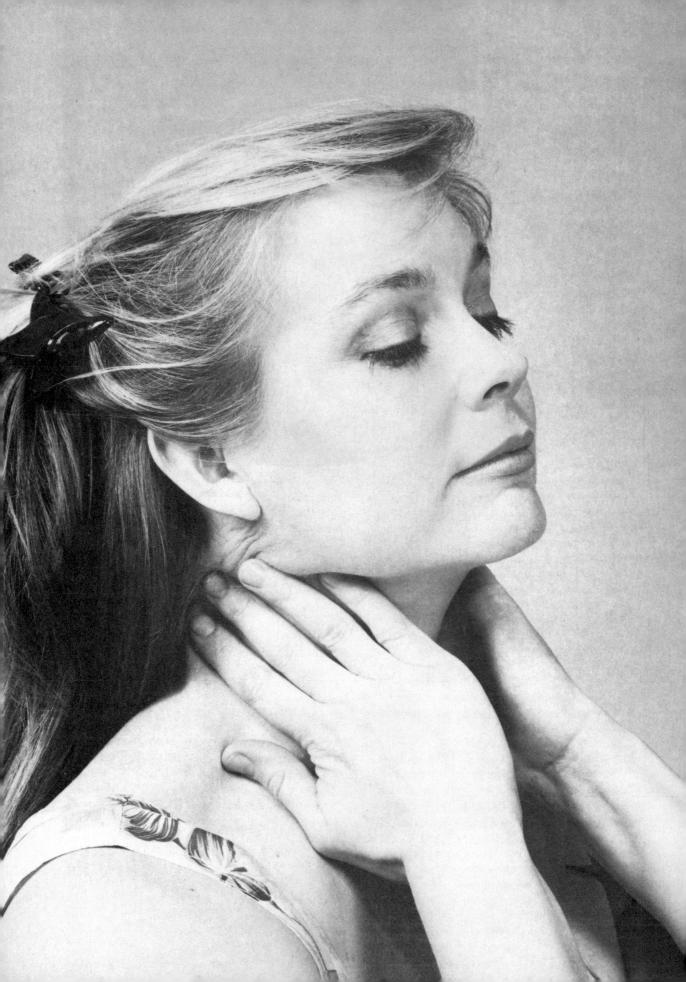

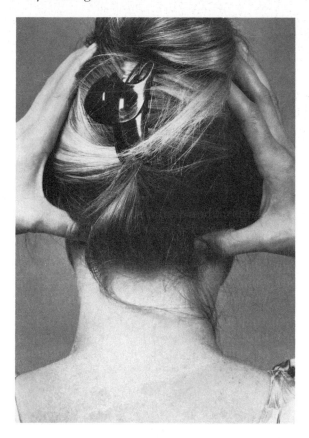

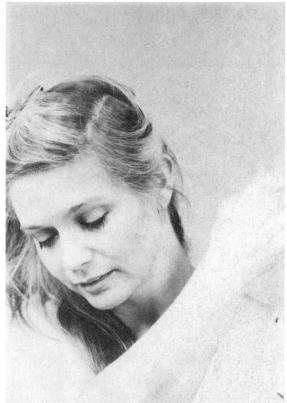

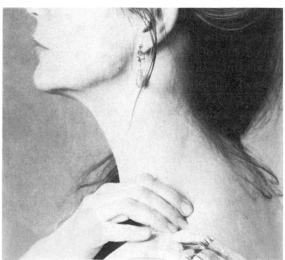

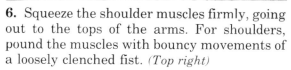

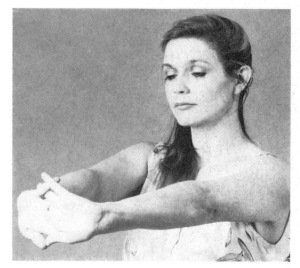

**6.** Squeeze the shoulder muscles firmly, going out to the tops of the arms. For shoulders, pound the muscles with bouncy movements of a loosely clenched fist. *(Top right)*

**7.** Press downwards at a spot halfway along the ridge of the shoulder muscle. Find the most painful spot to press, and you will be rewarded by a release of tension. *(Bottom left)*

**8.** Squeeze firmly down your arms from shoulder to wrist. Do it twice on each arm, so as to cover all the arm surface. Pound down each arm with a loosely clenched fist.

**9.** Massage your hands; rub the palm between the thumb and fingers of the other hand; pull and massage each finger; press firmly on the web of flesh between thumb and forefinger. Interlock fingers and stretch arms out with palms facing away from you. *(Bottom right)*

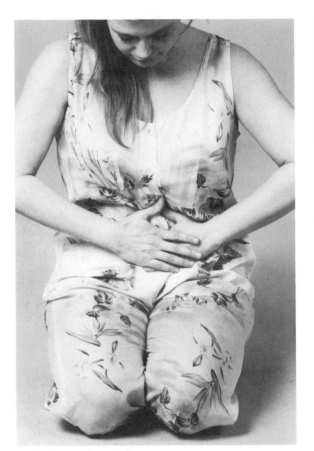

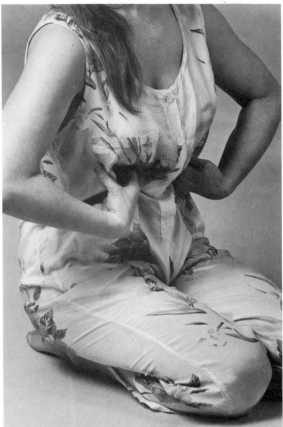

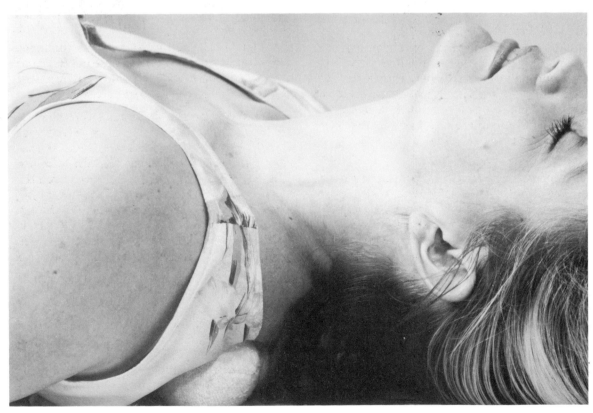

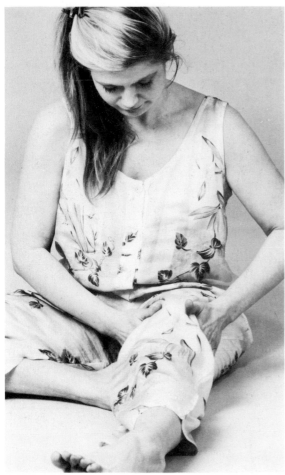

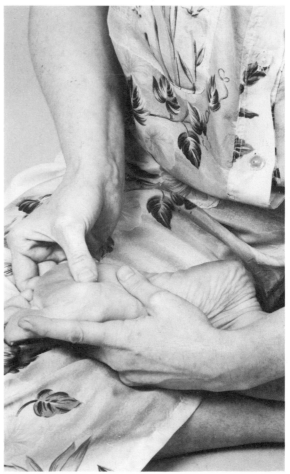

**10.** Massaging the Hara, or abdomen, is a great way to maintain a healthy digestion. With one hand on the other, rotate the soft tissues of your belly in a clockwise direction several times (up to 50 for maximum effect). Press deeply enough to feel it in your digestive organs as you rotate. *(Opposite top left)*

**11.** A good movement to improve the tone of the bowel is to kneel and place your fingers under your ribcage, pointing in to your belly. Breathe in, and as you exhale bend slowly forwards, so tnat your fingers are driven deep into your stomach. *(Opposite top right)*

**12.** Massaging your own back is hard to do. I find the most relaxing thing is to place my fists on either side of my spine and then to lie on them. You can get the same result from two rubber balls knotted into a sock to keep them at the correct distance apart. Place the balls on the ground and lie on them in such a way that they press on each side of your spine in the

shoulder area. Then move them so that they press a little further down, and so on. Roll your body to adjust the balls so that they massage you where needed. *((Opposite bottom)*

**13.** The legs are the easiest area on which to use long stroking movements, but pull up your legs rather than stroking down them, so that you help the circulation along. I find that for relieving tension it is more effective to roll the muscles of my thigh and calf vigorously between my palms, moving up and down the leg. You have to be sitting on the floor or a bed to do this, with your legs stretched out and relaxed. Pounding down the legs with a loosely clenched fist is stimulating. *(Above left)*

**14.** If you can put your foot on your knee, sole upward, it is easy to massage your own feet. Press with little rotary movements of your thumbs over the whole surface of the foot, sides and top as well as sole. If you cannot put your foot on your knee, try sliding your fingertips under your foot as it rests on the floor. *(Above right)*

# Checklist for Complete Body Massage

## Back

1. Effleurage
2. Petrissage up one side of back, across shoulders and down other side
3. Effleurage
4. Circular frictions up sides of spine
5. Effleurage
6. Percussion (optional)
7. Effleurage
8. Featherlight stroking

## Back of Legs

1. Effleurage
2. Petrissage on calf
3. Petrissage on thigh in three sections
4. Press-slide on sides of thigh
5. Effleurage

Your partner now turns over

## Front of legs

1. Effleurage
2. Half-and-half effleurage up shin
3. Grasp-slide on knee
4. Petrissage on thigh in three sections
5. Press-slide on sides of thigh
6. Effleurage
7. Clasp hands over top of foot, work on sole with thumbs
8. Effleurage over whole leg

## Abdomen

1. Circular effleurage
2. Effleurage up ribs, round sides to back, down towards groin
3. Petrissage on sides of hips and waist
4. Repeat effleurage 1 and 2

## Arms

1. Effleurage
2. Open hands to work on palm
3. Pump, stroke and rotate fingers
4. Effleurage

## Chest and Neck

1. Effleurage across chest, round back of shoulders and up back of neck
2. Rotary movements up back of neck
3. Repeat effleurage

## Face and Head

1. Stroke face from centre out towards ears
2. Stroke forehead
3. Pinch eyebrows
4. Circle eyes
5. Massage ears
6. Rake fingers through hair

# Now read on

Monika Struna and Connie Church, **Self Massage** (Hutchinson, 1983)

George Downing, **The Massage Book** (Wildwood House, 1973)

Tina Heinl, **Baby Massage** (Prentice Hall, 1983)

Eunice D. Ingham, **Stories that Feet can Tell Thru Reflexology, Stories that Feet have Told Thru Reflexology** (Ingham Publishing, 1984)

Lucy Lidell and others, **The Book of Massage** (Ebury Press, 1984)

Wataru Ohashi, **Do-it-yourself-Shiatsu** (Unwin Paperbacks, 1976)

Shirley Price, **Practical Aromatherapy** (Thorsons, 1985)

Maggie Tisserand, **Aromatherapy for Women** (Thorsons, 1985)

Robert Tisserand, **The Art of Aromatherapy** (C.W. Danicl, 1977)

J. Valnet, **The Practice of Aromatherapy** (C.W. Daniel, 1982)

## About the author

Carola Beresford-Cooke was brought up in the Far East. She returned to England to complete her education at St. Paul's Girl's School and St. Anne's College, Oxford. She began studying massage in 1975, and has been working at it professionally ever since.

Her areas of interest are Aromatherapy and Shiatsu. It was to further her understanding of oriental medical theory that she began to study acupuncture, and she is now a qualified acupuncturist. She prefers, however, to work with her hands rather than with needles. She teaches and lectures on massage and Shiatsu, and has a full-time massage practice in London.

## Acknowledgements

Thanks to Ondine, Margaret and Hazel for optimism and peppermint tea when I needed it most; to Deirdre Headon for her editorial labours; to Brian Inglis for his constant support. Finally to John Steele for inspiration on aromatherapy and for boosting my self-confidence all along.

And special thanks to all the models: Sarah Eagleton, Sherrie Dingle, Val Dozmary, Dawn Galton, Roger Galton, John Gibson, Sylvia Goodwin, Lesley Hilton, Georgia Robinson, Daisy Sutherland, Jane Thomas and Richard Van Spall.

# INDEX